AYURVEDA

INSPIRED COOKING FOR YOUR INDIVIDUAL WELL BEING

by Anne Bühring and Petra Räther

Photography by Heinz-Josef Beckers

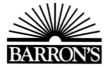

BARRON'S

CONTENTS

3

What Is Ayurveda?

The term *Ayurveda* comes from the ancient Indian Sanskrit: *ayus* means "life," and *veda* means "complete knowledge." So *Ayurveda* is "the knowledge of life." According to the self-concept of Ayurveda, this complete knowledge of life is a timeless reality, namely the laws of nature, which have been in effect everywhere since the beginning of creation. This knowledge of life is rooted in the consciousness of every person. The wise seers of the ancient Vedic high culture of India, the so-called *rishis*, have recognized these natural laws through introspection, and have passed on their knowledge orally from generation to generation. The oldest writings are dated from the third millennium to the eighth century B.C. Therefore, the Ayurveda is the oldest-known health teaching and is termed "the mother of medicine."

Maharishi Ayurveda

Several years ago, through the initiative of Maharishi Mahesh Yogi, this knowledge was introduced to the Western world and combined with modern science. This complete Ayurveda, which has become almost exclusively applied in the West, has become known as the Maharishi Ayurveda, and embraces more than twenty different formulations for perfect health: for example, advice for the daily routine, body care and diet, food supplements, aroma therapy, methods of purification, music therapy, meditation, and body and breathing exercises.

The Art of Ayurvedic Cooking

A central theme is the diet. The Ayurveda recognizes each human being as unique and having different requirements. The goal is to recognize what is good and healthy for you, for tastes are different. What is suitable for one, may not be right for another. Your body knows precisely what it needs. A kind of "physical intelligence" enables us to choose exactly the right foods from a multitude of offerings— in an entirely natural way. In modern times, however, this physical intelligence in all of us has become overshadowed by wrong eating habits, societal pressures, and stress.

About this Book

This cookbook gives you the chance to rediscover your physical intelligence. First take the test beginning on page 8 and find out which *dosha* (aspect of the physical intelligence) is dominant in you. In the test interpretation, you will learn tips and suggestions appropriate to your dosha dominance.

You can vary the recipes you find (beginning on page 22) according to your type, in order to harmonize your dosha dominance. Generally, this can be done easily for one or two people. If it is too much trouble—especially if you are cooking for several people with different dominants—you can simply prepare the dish for taste.

We offer additional Ayurvedic advice for practical conversion in the introductory text to each chapter.

The recipes are suitable for introduction to beginners, but they also offer new ideas for those familiar with Ayurvedic cuisine. They are typically Indian, but fit Western tastes, using spices and vegetables that are readily available.

An overview of the most important spices is listed on pages 38 and 39.

Appropriate for Vegetarians

The Ayurveda recognizes nonvegetarian dishes. However, it considers red meat very difficult to digest, and only suitable for people who have a certain constitution, perform hard physical labor, and, at the same time, have very good digestion.

In the spirit of the Ayurveda, we hope that this book helps you rediscover yourself and your needs—for comfort, good health, and inner happiness.

Cooking Ayurvedic

The recipes on the following pages are portioned for two people. You can halve or double them as necessary. You can harmonize your dosha dominance (see "Harmonizing Your Dosha Dominance") with the variations at the end of each recipe.

On page 57 you will find some tips on cooking for several people.

A Special Note:

The nutritional charts are provided for the original recipes only—not for the individual doshas. The nutrition information is approximate. The quantity of salt, if not specified, used for the analyses is $^{1}/_{8}$ of a teaspoon.

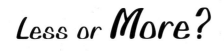

Less or **More?**

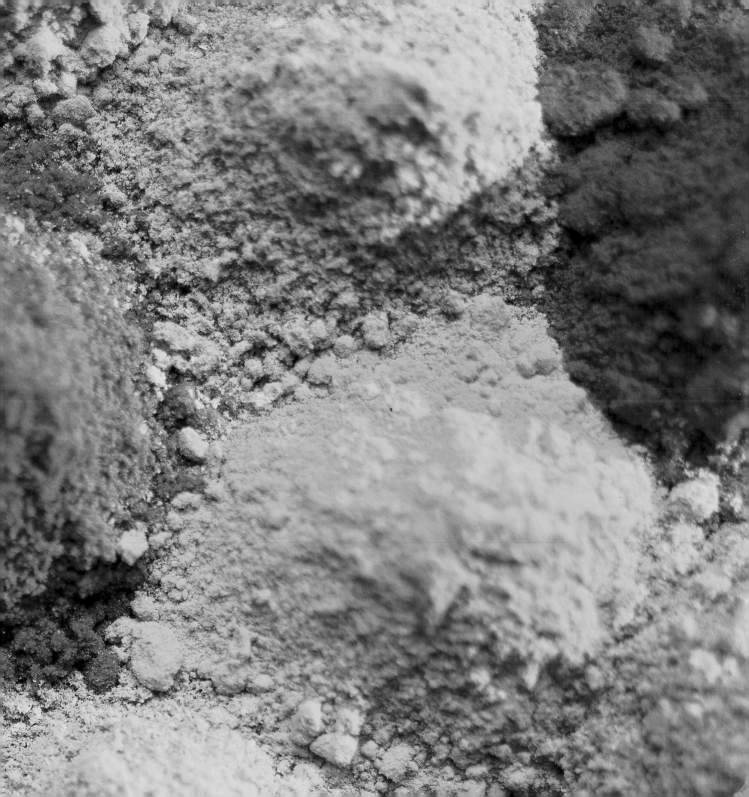

The Dosha Dominance

Vata, Pitta, Kapha

The doshas are basic functioning principles of which all creation is composed:

Vata— represents the elements air and space

Pitta— represents the fire element

Kapha— represents the elements water and earth

From these elements it can easily be deduced which characteristics are attributed to the doshas, for example:

Vata— airy-light, dry, cold, raw

Pitta— fiery-hot, sharp, slightly moist

Kapha— heavy, cold, soft, sticky, sweet

Imagine a crispbread: It is light, crispy-dry, and cold. Although all three doshas are present in crispbreads, the characteristics of Vata predominate. A fire-red chile pepper, on the other hand, very obviously has a high Pitta portion, and cold, sweet milk pudding is representative of Kapha. All three doshas also work in our bodies, but the ratios in which they work are unique to each individual. Thus, many personalities arise. If you know which dosha is dominant in you, you can recognize more easily which foods are good for you and which are not. The foods and drinks that balance, or harmonize, your dosha dominance will be soothing.

This means that we would not give a "hothead" with Pitta dominance fiery chile peppers, but rather something cooling. This way his Pitta will be balanced. The chile pepper is better suited to a Kapha type because it gives him enough fire and incentive to balance his heaviness (see food tables on the back flaps).

Dosha Test

This test is a simplified opportunity to determine your dosha dominance. For a detailed dosha analysis or in illness, see an Ayurvedic physician for a pulse diagnosis (see page 39 for an address to write away for more information).

Vata Test

Questions	Doesn't apply				Applies
	0	1	2	3	4
1. My body build is light. Joints and veins are prominent.					
2. I move and act fast.					
3. I gain weight with difficulty.					
4. My skin is tender and rather rough and dry.					
5. I sleep lightly, with interruptions, often sleeping badly.					
6. I have an irregular appetite and eat irregularly.					
7. I find cold weather unpleasant.					
8. I quickly take up something new, and also quickly forget it again.					
9. It is difficult for me to make decisions.					
10. I am lively and creative.					
11. I am slightly anxious, worry, and think a lot about things.					
12. I am alert and talkative.					
13. In stressful situations, I am easily excited.					
14. I have a tendency to be constipated and bloated.					
15. I have slightly cold hands and feet.					

Total points:

With this test you can easily establish which of the three doshas—Vata, Pitta, Kapha— is dominant in you. The test is divided into three areas of questions. Read the statements for the Vata first, then the Pitta, and finally the Kapha.

Decide how precisely each statement describes you, then choose the values of 0–4 as appropriate.
0 = doesn't apply
4 = applies

After scoring each section, total the number of points. In the right-hand column on page 11 you can read how to grade the three scores. The interpretations starting on page 12 will help you understand the doshas. You can then prepare the recipes that balance your dosha dominance. Thus, your body and soul will be in harmony with your nature.

Pitta Test

Questions	Doesn't apply				Applies
	0	1	2	3	4
1. I have a moderately heavy body build.					
2. I move and act forcefully and precisely.					
3. I can eat a lot and digest well.					
4. My skin is soft and rather pinkish with freckles.					
5. I have fine hair and tend to early graying and hair loss.					
6. I have a big appetite and am irritated if I don't get anything to eat.					
7. In hot weather, I feel uncomfortable.					
8. I can memorize well, and have a good memory.					
9. I am a perfectionist.					
10. I am quickly irritated or angered if things don't go the way I want them to.					
11. I have a keen mind.					
12. I am an impatient person.					
13. My work is precise and well organized.					
14. I sweat easily.					
15. I like ice cream and cool drinks.					

Total points:

Kapha Test

Questions	Doesn't apply				Applies
	0	1	2	3	4
1. My body build is heavy and muscular.					
2. I move and act slowly and steadily.					
3. I gain weight easily, tend to be overweight.					
4. My skin is soft, tough, and rather oily.					
5. I sleep long, deeply, and soundly.					
6. I can easily skip a meal if I am busy.					
7. Cold, damp weather is my least favorite.					
8. I have a very good long-term memory.					
9. I am even-tempered and calm.					
10. I have a tendency to be lazy.					
11. I am a peaceful person, and am hard to get riled up.					
12. I go about things slowly and quietly but with great perseverance.					
13. Routine situations make me contented; I like my "comfort zones."					
14. I have a tendency to be phlegmy, and have sensations of fullness.					
15. Wasting money isn't my problem; rather, I am too tight-fisted.					

Total points:

How You Establish the Dosha Dominance

You have responded to all three sets of statements and have added up the total points. Now determine in which dosha you have the most points; that will be your dominance. If the points of two doshas are very close together, it can indicate double dominance in your case; many people have double dominance. Next, read the comments in the right-hand columns on pages 13, 15, or 17.

There also are triple-dosha types, people who have all three points tallying very close together (page 17), but that is rare.

In the interpretations on the following pages, you will quickly recognize yourself; it isn't a matter of forcing yourself into a category. The dosha dominance serves as the first orientation with which you can trust your own needs and recognize what is right and healthy for you. This also applies to our recipes; here, too, you should listen to yourself, what you like, and what makes you feel good.

Interpretation: Vata Dominance

What is Vata?

Vata is the principle of movement. It is responsible for all transport and motion processes in the body. Vata consists of the elements of air and space. It controls growth, breath, blinking, and blood flow. It regulates the activity of the brain and causes alertness, clarity, and creativity. It is the pacemaker for all the bodily processes. The emotions of anxiety and fear are under the control of the Vata principle.

Vata has the qualities of dry, cold, rough, clear, light, and speed. Too much of it gets Vata out of balance. Substances that oppose those qualities calm Vata. People in whom Vata is dominant have a quick and alert mind, great flexibility, and are very creative. They are physically and mentally active. They have a light body build and low weight, often small shoulders or hips. Tendons, joints, and veins are very prominent. They have irregular appetites and usually put on weight with difficulty.

The basic mood of people with Vata dominance is mostly cheerful. They act quickly, are volatile, and are prone to forgetfulness. They have a pronounced dislike of cold and noise. Vata dominance makes people lively, talkative, imaginative. Food is preferred hot; cold is refused.

In Imbalance

With increased Vata, people tend to worry and think about things too much. Nervousness, anxiety, and sleeplessness are the results. Often, people with Vata dominance have dry skin. Since Vata increases with age, very dry skin can become a problem. Constipation, poor digestion, and bloating are typical for Vata imbalance, also back pain, menstruation problems, as well as cold hands and feet. In stress, Vata types easily exhaust themselves and do not make time for rest that is especially necessary for them.

What Does Good?

Sufficient rest and sleep are very important, as are regular daily routines with much warmth and rest breaks. The main theme is "regularity"—even if that is difficult for the active and jumpy Vata people. Mild exercise also has a positive effect. Divide your mental work so that you don't need to concentrate for too long. Try to avoid noise, perpetual conversation, and constant stimulation. A long bath in the morning and a friendly, warm environment harmonize any Vata dominance. Absolutely avoid fasting. For lack of food leads to a more severe increase of Vata, and will make you nervous and discontented. Drugs and too much sugar unbalance Vata. Quiet and meditation are especially soothing.

Eating

Regular meals and short periods without food are the cornerstones of the Vata diet. The Vata type should avoid cold foods as well as frozen and dried foods. Also, raw foods, especially lettuce and cabbage, are not well suited to Vata dominance. Bitter and sharp foods should be eaten less frequently. Warm meals and particular spices can harmonize Vata. Soups, hot drinks, rice with some butter or oil, cream of wheat, as well as milk drinks are good for Vata. Foods with sweet, salty, or sour tastes are especially beneficial. Tensions at the table will affect the Vata type's stomach, so it is especially important that you take your meals in a relaxed, quiet atmosphere.

You will find a detailed table with suitable foods on the back cover flap. In the recipes you should choose the variations for Vata.

Double Dominance

Vata-Pitta Dominance

Read both interpretations for Vata and Pitta dominance. You combine the dynamic of Pitta with the lightness of Vata, that is, you are alternatingly or concurrently under the influence of Vata and Pitta. Perhaps you also have noticed that you unite certain characteristics in yourself. For instance, you can react both anxiously and angrily in stressful situations. Or, you recognize that in summer you have more of a Pitta dominance, and in winter prefer Vata, since you are sensitive to cold.

In Vata-Pitta imbalance, a susceptibility to cardiac illness can be observed. In the recipe variations and food tables, you should read the recommendations for Vata and Pitta, and choose according to your taste.

Interpretation: Pitta Dominance

What Is Pitta?

Pitta is responsible for the metabolism. It comprises the elements of fire and water. The Pitta dosha controls digestion, metabolism, body temperature, intelligence, understanding, skin color, and the sparkle in the eye. Anger, hate, and jealousy are awakened by Pitta.

It has the qualities of hot, sharp, sour, slightly oily. Substances of this sort increase Pitta, opposites soothe this dosha.

People with Pitta dominance have a well-functioning metabolism, good digestion, and a strong urge for movement. Usually the body is slender but nevertheless muscular. Pitta promotes an alert mind, precise and clear speech, as well as a keen intellect. Much energy, strength of purpose, and willpower are typical. Pitta types understand superbly how to take responsibility for themselves, their lives, and their healing process. With Pitta dominance, early hair loss frequently occurs. The hair is usually fine or reddish, often graying early. Under stress, Pitta people tend to be critical, impatient, irritable, and have outbursts of rage. However, their basic mood is cheerful. Pitta people love order. They are enterprising, ambitious, and inventive. Most Pitta people are good talkers and organizers.

In Imbalance

When the pitta type is out of balance, he turns into a perfectionist. With too much self-criticism, impatience, and outbursts of rage, he makes life hard for himself (and others). On the physical side, reddened and sensitive skin, heartburn, and inflammations are recorded. With severe disturbances, common stress symptoms appear, and the danger of a heart attack increases. The first clear signs of an imbalance of Pitta are undisciplined appetite and gluttony.

What Does Good?

Maintaining calm and taking time for yourself and your hobbies are extremely important. The lead theme is "restraint." An excess of heat and steam (a sauna, for instance) should be avoided. In strong summer sun, you should protect your head, and on hot days, seek a cool place. However, you generally should stay in the fresh air. Don't shower in water that is too warm or dress too warmly. Too much sun, a hot climate, and sharp food irritates Pitta.

If you are feeling angry and compulsive, you should bring more self-control into your life. Step on the brakes, change your daily routine, and allow yourself more leisure time. You also need free time to enjoy beauty and nature.

Since coolness reduces Pitta, a cold compress on the forehead in stressful situations has a comforting effect.

Eating

Even if the Pitta type has an outstanding digestion and strong appetite, he should not eat too much. Sharp, salty, and sour foods, such as vinegar, ketchup, and sour cream, should be reduced, as these irritate Pitta. Don't eat too much salt, and eat few deep-fried foods. Also avoid coffee, alcohol, red meat, and sharp spices, such as chilies and cayenne pepper. Onions, garlic, tomatoes, and honey also are unfavorable; they have a heating effect.

Instead, choose foods with bitter, tart, and sweet flavors. Fresh fruits and vegetables, lots of milk and whole-wheat products should form the cornerstones of the menu. Lettuce, especially in summer, has a harmonizing effect. Grapes and pomegranates, as well as cooling dairy products, such as ghee and cream, also are recommended.

Refer to the detailed food tables for the Pitta type in the back cover. In the recipes, choose the variants for Pitta.

Double Dominance

Pitta-Kapha Dominance

Read both interpretations for Pitta and Kapha dominance. With a Pitta-Kapha dominance the influences of Pitta (dynamic) and Kapha (stability) are in effect alternately or simultaneously. In summer, you may have a Pitta dominance, and in spring a Kapha dominance, which could put you at risk for a Kapha imbalance. Or you may combine certain traits of Pitta and Kapha. This dosha combination often is found in athletes and people in leadership positions. In the recipe variations and food tables, check out the suggestions for Pitta and Kapha and choose according to your taste.

Interpretation: Kapha Dominance

What Is Kapha?

Kapha produces stability and permanence. This principle comprises the elements of earth and water. It keeps all the elements and structures in the body together, and it maintains the body's resistance. Kapha represents weight, stamina, mass, and fertility. It also influences the moisture of the skin and synovial fluid, and promotes wound healing, vitality, and stability.

The Kapha characteristics are heavy, cold, oily, soft, stable, and sweet.

Kapha people are down to earth and rely on their feelings. They have a strong stamina and react well to exercise. Their body build is rather stable-muscular. Out-of-balance Kapha people tend to be overweight, especially with excess fat on the legs and buttocks. They display patience and strength. The Kapha type carries out his plans slowly, with much thoughtfulness and certainty. Strong self-confidence allows him to be seldom upset. Patience,

stability, accommodation, generosity, and dependability are the chief characteristics of people with Kapha dominance. Also, if you love calm and permanence, a certain measure of change and movement can promote equilibrium.

In Imbalance

The desire to cling to old behavior patterns and rules can be so strong that it leads to rigidity and meanness. When the diet consists of too much heavy food, Kapha types tend to put on weight. Getting rid of excess pounds is especially important for Kapha people, because if they slip out of balance, they quickly become overweight. Tendency to oily skin and hair, depression, apathy, and lethargy are characteristic of Kapha disturbances. Kapha controls mucus production. In imbalance, diseases of the sinuses and colds are common. Abdominal distention, bronchitis, and diabetes are typical consequences of a Kapha imbalance.

What Does Good?

Much movement and change in life is good. The lead theme is "stimulation." Any stagnation leads to indolence and hinders further developmental processes. No one needs sports activity, variety, and change more than people with Kapha dominance. You should avoid sitting activities if possible. Dryness, warmth, and reduction of sugar consumption are important.

Eating

Basically the use of fats should be reduced, and deep-fried foods avoided. With a Kapha dominance, you also can fast over a long period of time, and thus, achieve a new quality of life.

As much as possible, Kapha types should reduce dishes that are sweet, sour, and salty. Most dairy products are unsuitable for Kapha: They only strengthen it. Small quantities of butter, oil, and sugar are tolerable.

You also should avoid cold drinks—warm water (see page 85) drunk throughout the day has a harmonizing effect.

Foods that are sharp, bitter, or tart are good. Warm, light, and dry foods, vegetables and herbs, and sharp, bitter, and tart spices are recommended. Large quantities of carbohydrates provide the active person with sufficient energy. It is important to finish the evening meal before sundown, and breakfast may be skipped entirely without concern. Raw foods are well tolerated, especially in summer, while warm casseroles and foods should be eaten in winter. In general, everything light and warm is good for Kapha.

For a choice of suitable foods, refer to the tables in the back cover for advice. In the recipes, choose the variations for Kapha.

Double Dominance

Kapha-Vata Dominance

Read the interpretations for Kapha and Vata dominance. You are alternately or concurrently under the influence of Vata (lightness) and Kapha (stability). Look at yourself to see what traits apply to you with regard to body build, reaction to stress, feelings or symptoms of imbalance. In any case, warmth is important for you.

With Kapha-Vata imbalance, a slow or irregular digestion may occur.

In the recipes and tables, read about Vata and Kapha, then choose according to availability and your tastes.

The Triple Dosha Type: Vata-Pitta-Kapha

Although quite rare, the Vata-Pitta-Kapha type has a good chance to stay in balance. You mostly enjoy good health, but must always pay attention to what is important for you! It is essential that you don't squeeze yourself into a category, but to be open to learn more about yourself.

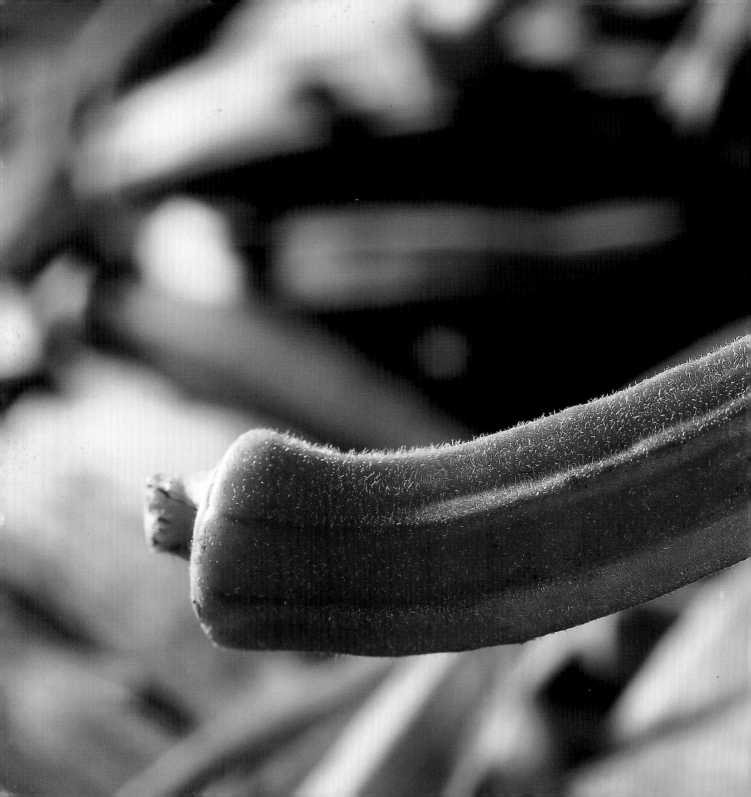

STARTERS

Appetizers and Salads

In the Ayurveda, one takes account of the digestive power of the stomach when planning the order of the menu, and so begins with the most difficult to digest, which are fried or raw foods, as well as very sweet things. You can begin with either a small portion of something sweet, a salad, or a grilled appetizer. Boiled food follows, and finally comes the lightest, perhaps a soup, if you are still hungry, or ripe fruit for dessert. In this chapter we have gathered some recipe ideas for appetizers.

Eating Tips

The Ayurveda attaches great importance to the appropriate diet. But it isn't only a matter of what you eat, but also when, where, and how the food is eaten. The following is a list of Ayurvedic eating recommendations:

• Eat in a calm and relaxed atmosphere. Consciously enjoy what you eat. Don't work or read while you eat. Sit down to eat, and when you can, eat at the same time every day—in as harmonious and relaxed a mood as possible.

• Don't eat too fast or too slowly. Eat until you are satisfied but not full (three-quarters of your satiation quantity is considered to be sufficient in the Ayurveda).

• Only eat when you are really hungry, that is, when your last meal is completely digested. After a main meal, wait three to six hours before eating again, with light meals wait one-half to two hours.

• You may drink something with your meal, but it should not be ice-cold. Water or lassi (see page 84) are appropriate, but not milk. Milk, as a drink, is only permitted with toast, wheat products, or sweet food, or about 20 minutes after the meal.

• After eating, stay at the table for a few minutes. Enjoy the relaxation before you resume your activities.

• It's best to prepare the food fresh—warm nothing up—and use the highest quality of ingredients. The most easily digested is warm, seasoned food with some fat.

Do You Go to Work?

If you eat your lunch in the office cafeteria, assemble your foods according to Ayurvedic criteria. Tip: Include some ghee, ginger, and your favorite spices or churnas (pages 38–39) to improve your food even further.

Can you not get any warm food at midday? Then perhaps you should consider carrying prepared food in a Thermos, or use a hot plate to prepare your food at work. In any case, a good lunch break should be a part of the working day! Your body will thank you for it.

Ghee—a Rasayana

Ghee (pronounced "gee," with a hard g) is similar to what we know as clarified butter. However, commercially prepared clarified butter contains chemical additives. Ghee is preferred over other fats for pan-frying and deep-frying, and can be added to food after cooking. For baking, however, use butter.

Ghee, along with milk and honey, is a naturally complete rasayana. Rasayanas strengthen the mind and body and work against the aging process, thus, ghee is suitable for any dosha dominance. Ghee makes food more digestible, intensifies the taste, and preserves the flavors in braising and sautéing. It also increases digestive activity without increasing Pitta.

Ghee can be bought in Indian grocery stores, but is easy to prepare at home. It keeps well and can be stored at room temperature. Ghee that has hardened will liquify again when warmed.

Preparing Ghee Yourself

• Melt several packages of unsalted butter in a deep pot over a low flame, and then allow the butter to simmer over low heat.

• During the next twenty to sixty minutes, depending on how much butter you are using, the water will evaporate, and a foam will develop on top. Do not stir or skim!

• Take the pot from the stove as soon as the foam has solidified and formed a light-brown crust on the bottom of the pot. Skim off the layer of foam on top, and carefully pour the clear ghee through a sieve lined with a paper towel or cloth into a heat-proof container. Throw away the deposits on the bottom.

• Good ghee is clear. If necessary, filter it again.

Fried Zucchini

4 oz (120 g) chickpea flour (available in health-food stores, Asian groceries)

salt

5 oz (150 ml) water

1¹/₈ lb (500 g) zucchini

5 oz (150 g) whole-milk yogurt

1 tablespoon corn oil

¹/₂ bunch mint

2 sprigs lemon balm

¹/₄ teaspoon ground cumin

For deep-frying:
1¹/₈ lb (500 g) ghee, or as needed

*Preparation time:
about 35 minutes
(+ 1¹/₂ hours resting time)*

Spinach Salad with Red Lentils

²/₃ lb (300 g) potatoes

salt

3¹/₂ oz (100 g) spinach leaves

1 cup (250 ml) vegetable broth

1³/₄ oz (50 g) red lentils

1 tablespoon ghee

¹/₂ cup (120 ml) water

¹/₂ bunch marjoram

¹/₄ teaspoon fenugreek seeds (page 39)

freshly ground black pepper

cayenne pepper

*Preparation time:
about 1 hour*

Fried Zucchini
Pictured

• In a large bowl, stir together the flour, salt, and water until smooth to make the batter. Let stand for about 1¹/₂ hours.

• Wash the zucchini, clean it, and slice about ¹/₂ inch (1¹/₂ cm) thick.

• Put yogurt and oil in a food processor. Remove and discard stems from mint and lemon balm leaves and add to the yogurt. Season with cumin, then process to purée.

• Lay the zucchini slices in the batter. Heat ghee in a wide pot or wok. Remove zucchini from the batter in portions and let drain a little. Carefully place zucchini slices in the hot ghee and fry 5 to 8 minutes, or until crispy brown. Repeat to fry all the zucchini. Serve.

Harmonize your dosha dominance:
Vata Add 1 teaspoon freshly grated ginger to the yogurt sauce.
Pitta Use olive oil or sunflower oil for the yogurt sauce. Instead of cumin, use ground coriander.
Kapha Not suitable, since it's fried.

PER SERVING:	535 CALORIES
NUTRITIONAL INFORMATION	
Carbohydrate 46	g
Protein 17	g
Total fat 39	g
Cholesterol 83	mg
Sodium 203	mg
Fiber 10	g

Spinach Salad with Red Lentils
Classic

• Cook the potatoes in a large pan of salted water for about 20 minutes, peel, and allow to cool. Wash and pick over the spinach, then let it drain.

• Bring the broth to a boil in a large pot and add the lentils; cook 10 to 15 minutes. Drain the lentils, reserving the broth. Mix the lentils and the spinach in a large serving bowl.

• Dice the potatoes and place them in a food processor with reserved broth; process to purée. In a small bowl, mix the ghee, water, and marjoram leaves; add to potato mixture. Grind the fenugreek seeds in a spice grinder then add to potatoes, along with pepper and cayenne; pour mixture over the spinach mixture. Makes 2 servings.

Harmonize your dosha dominance:
Vata Not suitable.
Pitta Prepare the salad without lentils. Instead of using cayenne pepper, season with ¹/₂ teaspoon each of coriander and turmeric. Enrich the potatoes with cream.
Kapha Very suitable without variations.

PER SERVING:	298 CALORIES
NUTRITIONAL INFORMATION	
Carbohydrate 51	g
Protein 12	g
Total fat 7	g
Cholesterol 16	mg
Sodium 241	mg
Fiber 12	g

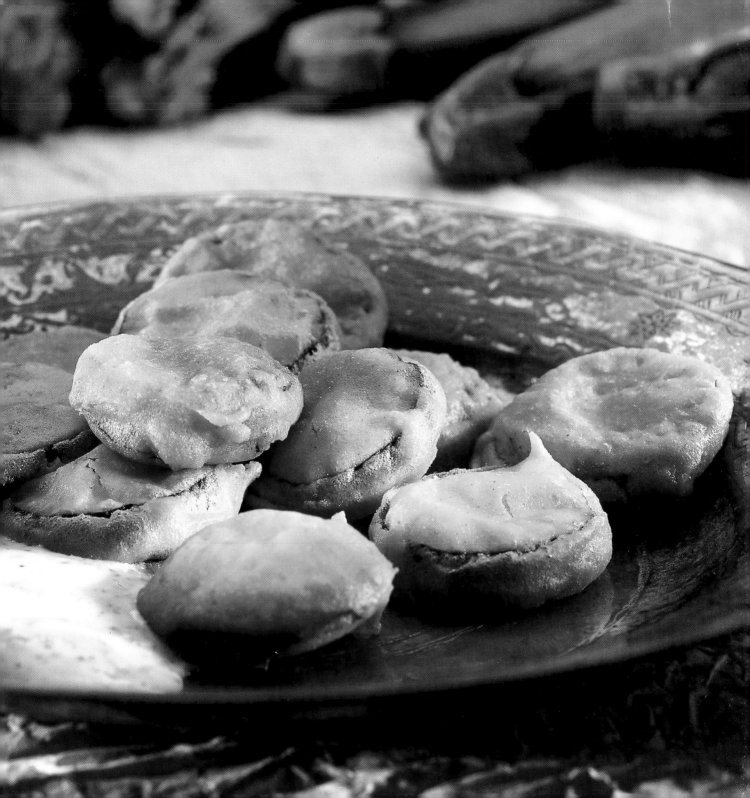

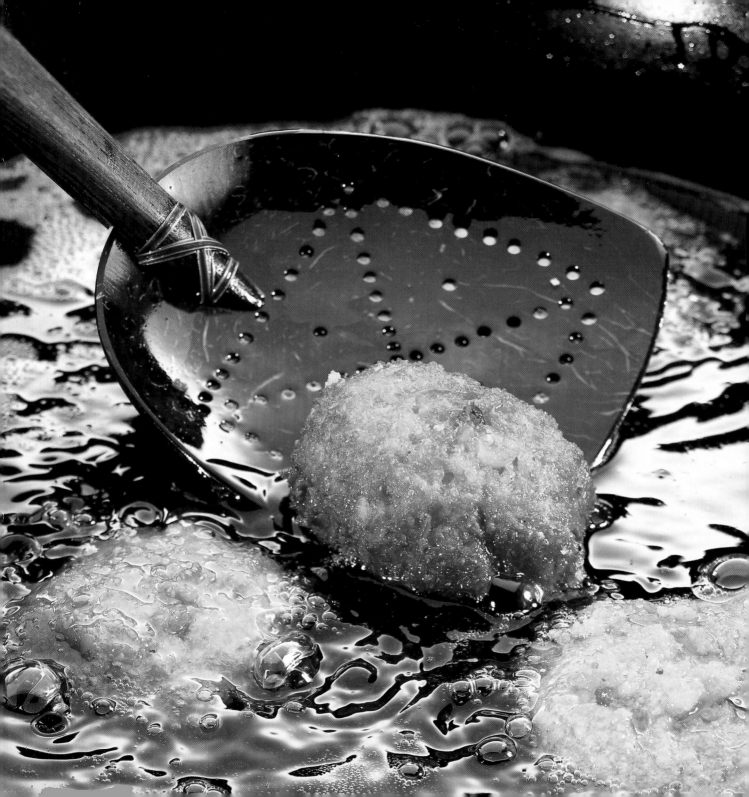

Pepper Salad
Easy to prepare

• Clean and seed the bell peppers, halve them, and cut into paper-thin slices. Grind the peppercorns in a spice grinder. Heat the oil in a pan and briefly sear the peppercorns and the cumin in it over medium heat. Add the nuts and continue to cook.

• Add the bell peppers and briefly cook without browning. Add the cream and let boil for a short time. Serve immediately with toast. Makes 2 servings.

Harmonize your dosha dominance:
Vata In addition, use $1/2$ teaspoon chopped basil or oregano.
Pitta Only use green bell peppers. Season with an additional $1/2$ teaspoon ground coriander and some turmeric.
Kapha Warm the vegetables in a little water for a short time, season to taste with freshly ground ginger; leave out the cream and nuts. Serve with crispbread.

Falafel with Herb Yogurt
Pictured

• Soften the peas overnight in plenty of cold water. Let drain, then purée in a food processor.

• Grind the spices in a spice grinder. Stir into the peas, along with the salt and flour; let stand about 3 hours.

• Beat the yogurt with 2 tablespoons water in a medium-size bowl. Stir in herbs, salt, and black pepper. Let stand in the refrigerator.

• Heat ghee. Using a tablespoon, drop spoonfuls of the pea mixture into the hot ghee; fry them crispy brown. Makes 2 servings.

Harmonize your dosha dominance:
Vata Instead of buckwheat, whole-wheat flour also is good. Serve warm.
Pitta Add black pepper to the falafel mixture.
Kapha Not suitable, since it is fried.

Pepper Salad

1 red bell pepper
$1/2$ yellow bell pepper
3 black peppercorns
2 tablespoons sunflower oil
$1/2$ teaspoon cumin seeds
$1^3/4$ teaspoons (50 g) cashews
2 tablespoons cream
2 slices whole-wheat toast

*Preparation time:
about 30 minutes*

Falafel with Herb Yogurt

For the falafel:
$1/3$ lb (150 g) dried split green peas
$1/4$ lb (100 g) dried split yellow peas
1 teaspoon each: coriander seeds, ground cumin, and salt
$2^1/2$ tablespoons (35 g) buckwheat flour

For the herb yogurt:
$2/3$ cup (150 g) whole-milk yogurt
2 tablespoons water
1 sprig tarragon, chopped
6 sprigs each, chopped: mint and lemon balm
salt
freshly ground black pepper

For frying:
$1^1/8$ lb (500 g) ghee, or more as needed

*Preparation time:
about 30 minutes
(+ softening time overnight
+ 3 hours steeping time)*

PER SERVING:		234 CALORIES
NUTRITIONAL INFORMATION		
Carbohydrate	17	g
Protein	4	g
Total fat	18	g
Cholesterol	6	mg
Sodium	140	mg
Fiber	4	g

PER SERVING:		383 CALORIES
NUTRITIONAL INFORMATION		
Carbohydrate	38	g
Protein	14	g
Total fat	20	g
Cholesterol	54	mg
Sodium	61	mg
Fiber	12	g

Rice Fritters with Herb Dip

2$^1/_2$ tablespoons (50 g) basmati rice

salt

$^1/_2$ lb (200 g) carrots

2 tablespoons whole-wheat flour

2 teaspoons turmeric

6 tablespoons cream

freshly grated nutmeg

$^1/_4$ teaspoon ground coriander

$^1/_2$ teaspoon curry powder or churna (see page 39)

2 tablespoons ghee

$^2/_3$ cup (150 g) whole-milk yogurt

1 bunch parsley

Preparation time: about 40 minutes

Okra Salad with Oranges

salt

$^1/_4$ lb (100 g) large white beans (canned)

$^1/_3$ lb (150 g) okra

2 oranges

2 tablespoons ghee

$^1/_2$ teaspoon fennel seeds

rock candy or sugar to taste

freshly ground black pepper

3 sprigs lemon balm

Preparation time: about 45 minutes

Rice Fritters with Herb Dip
Suitable for guests

• Cook the rice in $^1/_2$ cup (120 ml) salted water over low heat for about 15 minutes. Let drain in a sieve.

• Meanwhile, peel the carrots, wash, and grate them; add to the rice. Stir in the flour, turmeric, and cream to make a thick batter. Season with nutmeg, coriander, and curry powder or churna. Heat the ghee in a pan. With a tablespoon, drop spoonfuls of batter into the pan, press them flat, and fry over moderate heat for about 8 minutes, turning once. Drain on paper towels.

• Beat the yogurt in a food processor with some water. Wash the parsley and remove stems. Add parsley leaves to yogurt, and purée. Season to taste with salt, and serve with rice fritters. Makes 2 servings.

Harmonize your dosha dominance:
Vata Very appropriate without variations.
Pitta Season the yogurt dip with less salt, using plenty of freshly chopped herbs and mint.
Kapha Eat only a few rice fritters without the dip. Use rye flour for the batter, and season with ginger and turmeric.

PER SERVING:	354 CALORIES	
NUTRITIONAL INFORMATION		
Carbohydrate	36	g
Protein	8	g
Total fat	20	g
Cholesterol	59	mg
Sodium	257	mg
Fiber	5	g

Okra Salad with Oranges
Pictured

• Bring a large pot of salted water to a boil. Add the beans and cook 10 minutes; drain. Cut the stems off the okra pods. Halve the pods once lengthwise. Peel the oranges, including the thick, white pith, and cut the oranges into sections, reserving the juice.

• Heat the ghee in a pan. Add the fennel seeds and briefly brown. Add the orange juice and bring to a boil. Add okra, beans, and rock candy and let simmer for about 5 minutes. Season to taste with salt and pepper. Cut the lemon balm leaves into strips, and add to bean mixture, along with oranges; stir to heat throughout. Makes 2 servings.

Harmonize your dosha dominance:
Vata Don't use white beans, but add radishes to the salad. Serve warm.
Pitta Use sweet oranges.
Kapha Not suitable.

PER SERVING:	320 CALORIES	
NUTRITIONAL INFORMATION		
Carbohydrate	48	g
Protein	8	g
Total fat	13	g
Cholesterol	33	mg
Sodium	154	mg
Fiber	9	g

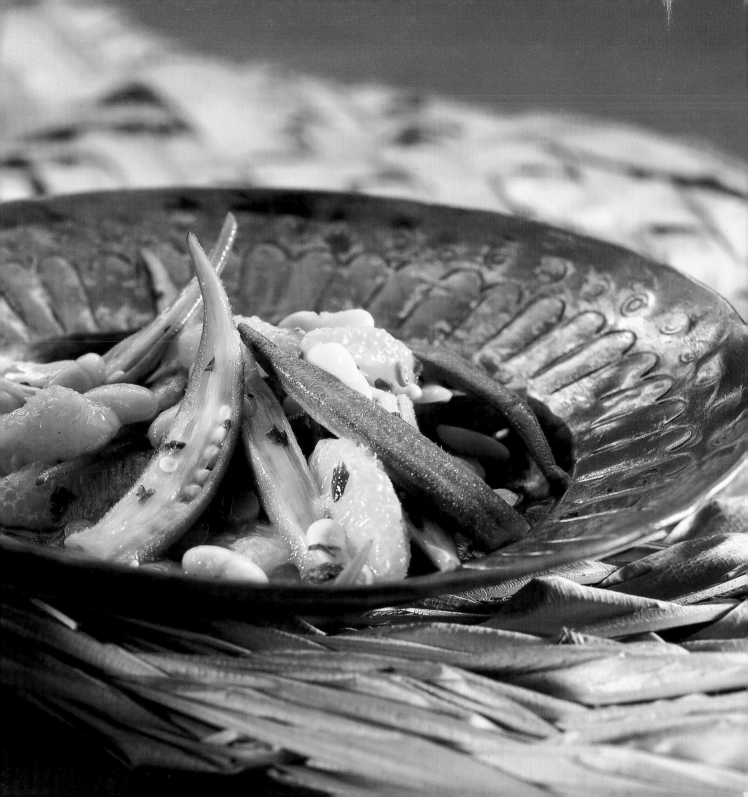

Broccoli with Lemon Marinade

salt

1¹/₈ lb (500 g) broccoli

3 black peppercorns

¹/₂ teaspoon coriander seeds

2 tablespoons fresh lemon juice

3 teaspoons sunflower oil

1 sprig cilantro

toasted whole-wheat bread

*Preparation time:
about 30 minutes*

Avocado Salad with Poori

For the poori (pancakes):

*¹/₂ cup plus 1 tablespoon
(125 g) whole-wheat flour*

*1¹/₂ to 2 tablespoons (50 g)
wheat flour*

¹/₄ teaspoon salt

¹/₄ teaspoon cumin

1 pinch of cayenne pepper

1 tablespoon ghee

*¹/₃ cup (75 ml) lukewarm
water*

For frying:

*1¹/₈ lb (500 g) ghee, or as
needed*

For the salad:

1 small avocado

2 to 3 tomatoes

fresh lemon juice

1 tablespoon olive oil

salt

freshly ground black pepper

*Preparation time:
about 40 minutes*

Broccoli with Lemon Marinade
Easy to Prepare

• Bring a large pot of salted water to a boil. Clean the broccoli, then peel the stems and cut into slices. Divide the head into small florets. Blanch the broccoli in the boiling water for about 5 minutes. Drain in a colander, then refresh under cold water.

• Grind peppercorns and coriander in a spice grinder. Combine peppercorn mixture and lemon juice in a large bowl. Add 1 pinch of salt, then beat in the oil. Add broccoli and toss to mix. Chop cilantro leaves and stir them in to broccoli mixture. Let stand for a short time. Serve with crisply toasted whole-wheat bread.

Harmonize your dosha dominance:
Vata Cabbage family vegetables are not suitable.
Pitta Use little lemon, or make a salad dressing without cream and oil; season with turmeric.
Kapha Serve lukewarm. Eliminate the salt, and season to taste with freshly grated ginger and nutmeg.

PER SERVING:	200 CALORIES	
NUTRITIONAL INFORMATION		
Carbohydrate	26	g
Protein	10	g
Total fat	9	g
Cholesterol	0	mg
Sodium	350	mg
Fiber	9	g

Avocado Salad with Poori
Pictured

• For the poori, mix both kinds of flour, salt, spices, and ghee in a large bowl. Slowly pour in the water, and knead into an elastic dough.

• In a large pot or wok, heat enough ghee for deep-frying. Divide the dough into six parts and form into balls. Brush your work surface with ghee, then roll each ball into a small pancake.

• When the ghee in the pan is very hot, turn down the heat; it should not smoke! Lay the pancakes in the ghee one at a time. When the dough puffs up, press it into the ghee with a skimmer until it blows up into a balloon; turn and cook a few seconds longer.

• Peel and dice the avocado. Wash the tomatoes, then seed and dice them. Place avocado and tomatoes in a serving bowl, then season with lemon juice, oil, salt, and pepper.

Harmonize your dosha dominance:
Vata Very suitable without variations.
Pitta Use avocado with additional herbs and only 1 tomato.
Kapha Not suitable.

PER SERVING:	529 CALORIES	
NUTRITIONAL INFORMATION		
Carbohydrate	46	g
Protein	9	g
Total fat	38	g
Cholesterol	34	mg
Sodium	468	mg
Fiber	13	g

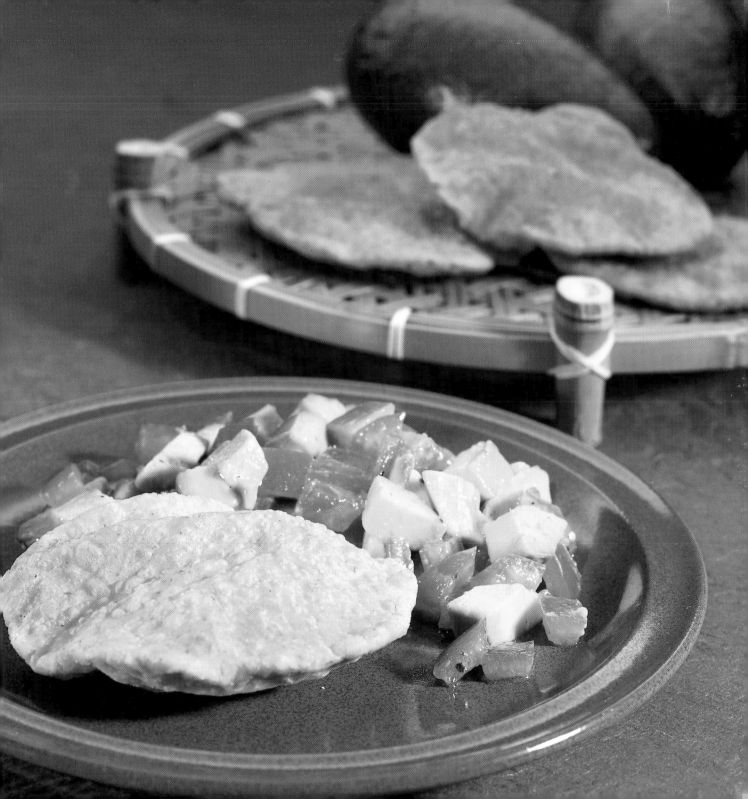

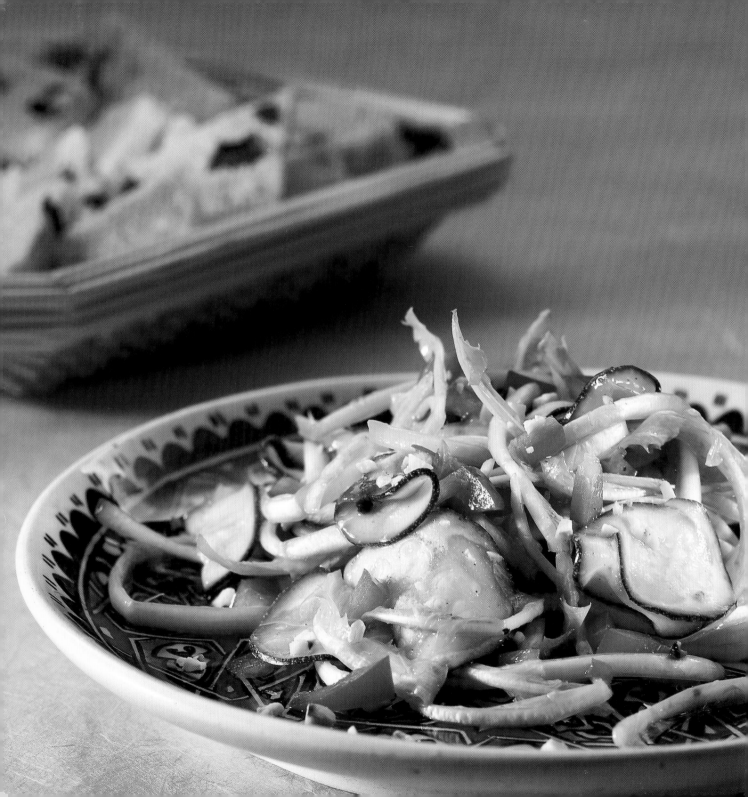

Dandelion Salad with Polenta
Pictured

• Heat the ghee in a large pan. Add cornmeal and cook over low heat. Add the broth, and stir until smooth; let stand for about 5 minutes. Fold in oregano. Grease a baking sheet, then spread the polenta in it evenly; let cool.

• Wash the vegetables. Dice the bell pepper very fine and place in a serving bowl. Slice zucchini thin and add to bowl. Tear dandelion greens into small pieces and add to bowl. In a small bowl, stir together the lemon juice, black pepper, coriander, and oil; toss with salad ingredients. Sprinkle nuts over the salad. Serve with polenta, cut into wedges. Makes 2 servings.

Harmonize your dosha dominance:
Vata Fry peppers and zucchini briefly in oil; add dandelion greens, and season. Serve lukewarm.
Pitta Use a green bell pepper. Substitute cream for the lemon juice in the dressing. Serve with toasted whole-wheat bread instead of the polenta.
Kapha Replace the cashews with sunflower seeds. Cook the cornmeal in broth, and add the ghee later.

PER SERVING:	462 CALORIES	
NUTRITIONAL INFORMATION		
Carbohydrate	49	g
Protein	8	g
Total fat	28	g
Cholesterol	16	mg
Sodium	77	mg
Fiber	7	g

Cauliflower–Broccoli Salad
Refreshing

• Bring a large pot of salted water to a boil. Soften diced prunes and raisins in a large bowl of cold water for several minutes, then drain. Divide cauliflower and broccoli into florets; blanch for about 3 minutes in the boiling water, then refresh in cold water; drain.

• In a large bowl, combine oil, lemon juice, and curry; mix well. Fold in the raisins and plums. Season with salt and pepper, then add cauliflower and broccoli, and toss to coat. Makes 2 servings.

Harmonize your dosha dominance:
Vata Not suitable.
Pitta Also season with coriander, fennel, or Pitta churna. Instead of lemon juice, use cream.
Kapha Season with ginger, turmeric, or Kapha churna. Use as little salt as possible.

PER SERVING:	412 CALORIES	
NUTRITIONAL INFORMATION		
Carbohydrate	46	g
Protein	7	g
Total fat	25	g
Cholesterol	0	mg
Sodium	200	mg
Fiber	7	g

Dandelion Salad with Polenta

1 tablespoon ghee
scant $1/2$ cup (100 g) cornmeal
1 scant cup (200 ml) vegetable broth
leaves from $1/2$ bunch oregano
1 red bell pepper
2 small zucchini
1 scant cup (100 g) dandelion greens
2 tablespoons fresh lemon juice
freshly ground black pepper
ground coriander
2 tablespoons sunflower oil
$3^1/2$ tablespoons cashews, toasted

For the baking sheet: oil

Preparation time: 50 to 60 minutes

Cauliflower–Broccoli Salad

salt
6 pitted prunes, diced
1 tablespoon raisins
$1/2$ small head cauliflower
$2/3$ lb (300 g) broccoli
$3^1/2$ tablespoons (50 ml) sunflower oil
fresh lemon juice to taste
1 teaspoon curry powder or churna (see page 39)
freshly ground black pepper

Preparation time: about 25 minutes

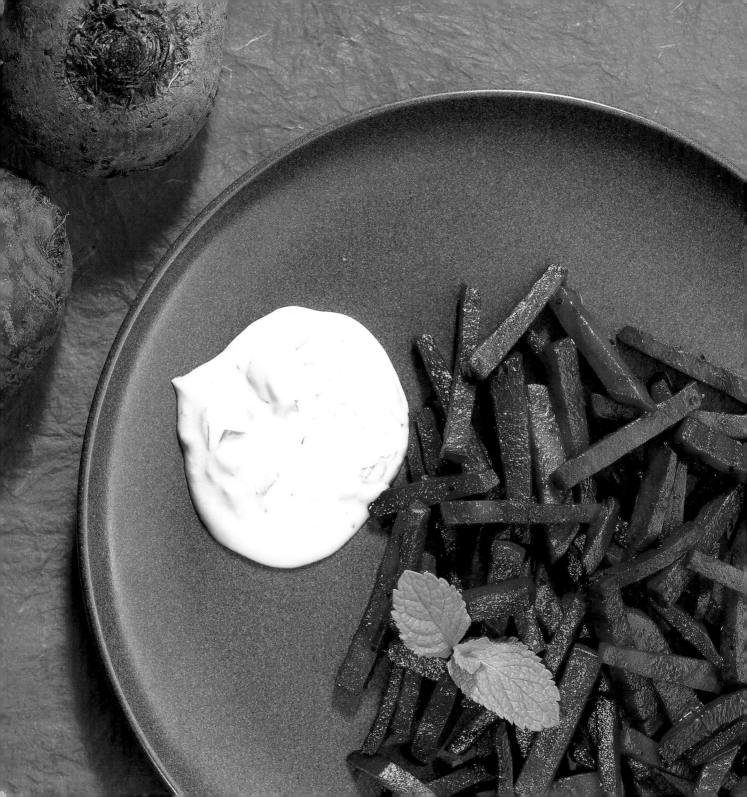

Mixed Salad
Refreshing

• Clean and seed bell peppers; dice small. Dice the cucumber. Cut the stems from each tomato; cut each tomato into eighths, and remove seeds. Chop the tarragon leaves.

• Heat the ghee in a pan; add the herbes de Provence and briefly heat. Add the lemon juice, and let come to a boil; toss in the vegetables and simmer briefly. Season with salt and pepper, then stir in the tarragon. Makes 2 servings.

Harmonize your dosha dominance:
Vata Serve lukewarm. Fry $1/2$ teaspoon of cumin seeds in ghee, and add along with the herbes de Provence.
Pitta Instead of red peppers, use endive. Use less tomato, and stir in mixed chopped fresh herbs. Substitute cream for the lemon juice.
Kapha Instead of cucumber, use leaf lettuce or sprouts. Don't heat the vegetables in the ghee, but dress them with lemon juice and sunflower oil. Season with ginger, turmeric, and black pepper.

Beets with Mint Yogurt
Pictured

• Peel beets under running water; cut into slices about $1/4$ inch ($1/2$ cm) thick, then cut into sticks.

• Heat the ghee in a pan. Add beets and cook over high heat until crispy, then cover and let braise over moderate heat for about 20 minutes. Season with salt and pepper.

• Chop mint leaves fine. Beat the yogurt in a small bowl with some water until creamy; stir in the mint. Season to taste with salt and pepper. Serve yogurt dressing with the warm beets. Makes 2 servings.

Harmonize your dosha dominance:
Vata In addition, cook $1/2$ teaspoon of black mustard seeds in the ghee until they burst, then add the beets.
Pitta Instead of beets, briefly fry zucchini slices in the ghee, and season with some coriander or churna.
Kapha Not suitable. Better to eat a raw beet salad.

Mixed Salad

1 red bell pepper
$1/2$ each green and yellow bell peppers
$1/4$ cucumber
2 tomatoes
1 bunch tarragon
2 tablespoons ghee
1 teaspoon herbes de Provence
2 teaspoons fresh lemon juice
salt
freshly ground black pepper

Preparation time: about 25 minutes

Beets with Mint Yogurt

2 small beets
2 tablespoons ghee
salt
freshly ground black pepper
a few sprigs of mint
$2/3$ cup (150 g) whole-milk yogurt

Preparation time: about 45 minutes

PER SERVING:	199 CALORIES	
NUTRITIONAL INFORMATION		
Carbohydrate	22	g
Protein	3	g
Total fat	13	g
Cholesterol	33	mg
Sodium	163	mg
Fiber	5	g

PER SERVING:	261 CALORIES	
NUTRITIONAL INFORMATION		
Carbohydrate	28	g
Protein	6	g
Total fat	15	g
Cholesterol	42	mg
Sodium	359	mg
Fiber	8	g

Endive-Pepper Salad with Chapati

For the chapati:

$1/2$ cup plus 1 tablespoon
(125 g) sifted whole-wheat
flour

$1/4$ teaspoon salt

$1/4$ cup plus 1 tablespoon
(75 ml) lukewarm water

2 tablespoons ghee

For the salad:

$1/2$ head green endive lettuce

$1/2$ each yellow and green
bell peppers

$1/4$ cucumber

$1/4$ teaspoon fennel seeds

$1/4$ teaspoon coriander seeds

3 black peppercorns

1 tablespoon ghee

2 tablespoons fresh lemon
juice

For dusting: flour

*Preparation time:
about 40 minutes
(+ 2 hours resting time)*

Endive-Pepper Salad with Chapati
More time-consuming

• For the chapati, mix flour and salt in a large bowl. Slowly add water. Knead until a soft dough develops. Lay the dough on a work surface and knead for 5 minutes more; the dough must be smooth and elastic. Dampen the dough ball with some water. Wrap in a dampened dish towel and set aside for about 2 hours (not in the refrigerator).

• Place a shallow cast-iron pan or crêpe pan over medium heat. Knead the dough once more, then divide into six pieces. Dust each piece with flour, then roll out each piece to about 6 inches (15 cm) in diameter. Shake off any excess flour. Place dough rounds in the pan and brown on both sides, pressing flat with a spatula; this may need to be done in batches. Wrap chapati in a kitchen towel to keep warm.

• For the salad, wash escarole and cut into bite-size pieces. Clean and seed the peppers, then slice paper thin. Cut the cucumber into small dice.

• Grind the fennel, coriander, and peppercorns together in a spice grinder.

Heat 1 tablespoon ghee in a pan over medium heat. Add spices and sauté until fragrant. Deglaze the pan with lemon juice, then add the prepared vegetables and toss briefly. Brush chapati with remaining 2 tablespoons ghee and pass with the salad.

Harmonize your dosha dominance:
Vata Instead of bell peppers, use radishes. Cook the salad somewhat longer and serve warm.
Pitta For deglazing, use cream instead of lemon juice.
Kapha Instead of cucumber, use radishes or celery. Season the salad with ginger, turmeric, and black pepper. Serve warm.

Tips:
Let the rolled-out chapati rest for a while, wrapped in a dish towel; they will fry better.
If you like the chapati rather crisp, cook them until they have numerous dark spots; with less cooking time, they are more elastic.

PER SERVING:	306 CALORIES	
NUTRITIONAL INFORMATION		
Carbohydrate 32	g
Protein 6	g
Total fat 19	g
Cholesterol 49	mg
Sodium 158	mg
Fiber 7	g

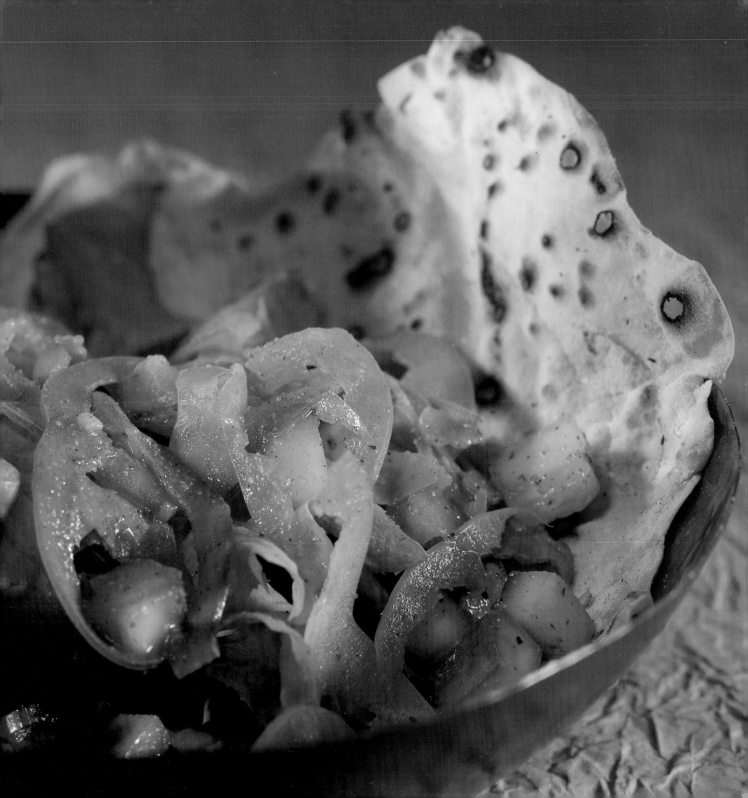

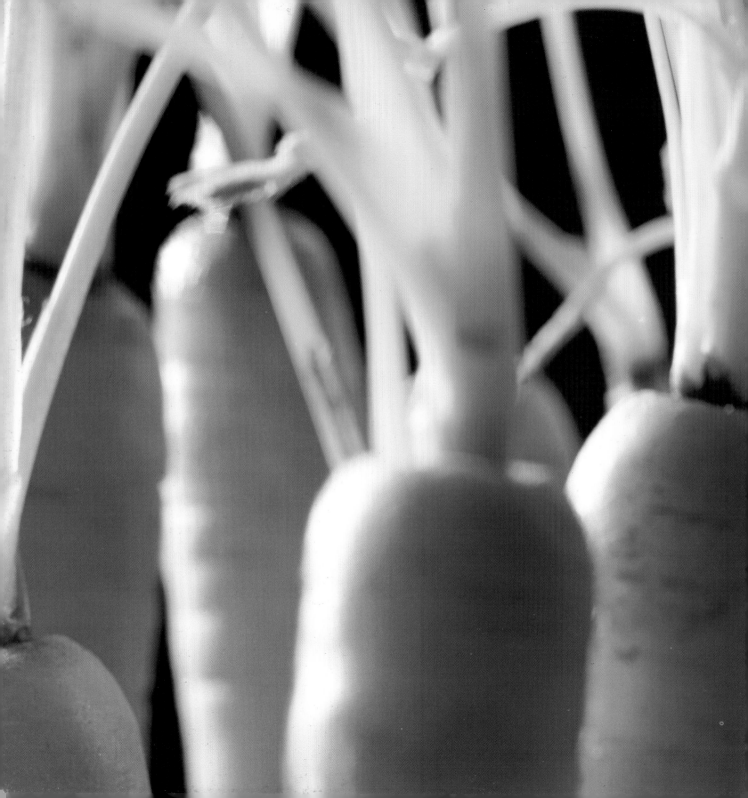

HIGH
POINTS

Braised Dishes and Curries

Spices play an important role that is not limited to the preparation of curries. Spices make food tastier and more easily digestible, and can change the dosha-specific effect of any dish.

In order to release their taste and full aroma, spices often are seared in a hot pan. It is important not to let them burn. Whole seeds, such as cumin and fennel, need about 30 seconds to brown; freshly grated ginger, about 20 seconds. Ground spices, such as coriander and turmeric, need a very short time, about 3 seconds. In general, other seasonings, such as lemon, salt, cream, or fresh herbs, are added at the end of cooking.

It pays to buy the spices whole, then grind or grate them before you use them, because the flavor is much more prominent.

The quantity of spices used is not determined by strict rules, but depends on your own taste. Although Ayurvedic food is always seasoned, it need not necessarily be hot. If you don't have a spice that your recipe calls for, you can substitute another spice, or leave it out, without the dish losing its taste.

The Important Spices

• Asafetida—is an aromatic gum that grows mainly in Iran and India. It can be found powdered or in lump form in Indian and Middle Eastern markets. It has a distinctive taste and odor, and should only be used in small quantities. If you can't get asafetida, your dish will taste fine without it. Asafetida also is used to break down the indigestible enzyme found in beans and vegetables of the cruciferous family.

• Black mustard seeds—are smaller than the yellow variety and are dark brown. You usually can find them in Asian stores and health-food stores. When they are seared in fat, they are done as soon as they begin to burst and jump; don't let them burn!

• Black onion seeds—also called nigella seeds, resemble, but are not true onion seeds. These tiny angular seeds have a nutty, peppery flavor. They can be found in Middle Eastern and Indian markets.

• Cardamom—the small green pods are used frequently for sweet dishes. You can cook with the entire pod or the small seeds inside. In the supermarket, you usually will find ground cardamom, which is less flavorful than freshly ground seeds.

• Coriander—the seeds and leaves of this plant in the parsley family are readily used. Coriander seeds are available whole and ground; the aromatic seeds release their best aroma and taste when freshly ground. The leaves, better known as cilantro or Chinese parsley, are used as frequently in East Indian cooking as parsley is in the United States. Coriander and cilantro are readily available in most markets. You also can grow the plant from the seeds.

• Cumin—is used whole or ground. It is a relative of caraway. Cumin is available in the spice section of most grocery stores.

• Fennel seeds—are used whole or ground. They can be found in most grocery stores. You also can substitute the same amount of anise seeds in a recipe calling for fennel seeds.

• Fenugreek seeds—are small, square, beige seeds with a pungent, slightly bitter taste. Use them sparingly, and don't let them burn. Fenugreek seeds can be bought whole or ground in health-food stores and Asian groceries. A native of Asia and southern Europe, fresh fenugreek is not generally available in the United States.

• Ginger—fresh or ground, is used often. Ground ginger can be bought in the supermarket; fresh ginger, a light-brown root, is available in most produce sections. Fresh ginger should be peeled before using, then chopped fine or finely grated. The powder is hotter than the fresh root; 1 teaspoon of ground ginger equals about 1 tablespoon of freshly grated ginger.

• Gomashio—Available in health-food stores and some Asian markets, gomashio is a seasoning composed of sea salt and toasted sesame seeds.

• Sambal oeleck—is a mixture of chilies, brown sugar, and salt that is used as a multipurpose condiment; it can be found in Asian markets.

• Turmeric—is the root of a tropical plant related to ginger. It gives food an intense yellow-orange color. You can find turmeric in supermarkets.

Churnas—One for Every Dosha

Vata, Pitta, and Kapha churnas are mixtures of spices that are tailored for each dosha dominance.

Seasoning with churnas is a simple and comfortable way for the Ayurveda fan to improve the food and adjust it to his taste and the dosha dominance. Churnas are available in selected health-food stores and from mail-order companies, as well as from the Maharishi Ayurveda Health Centers. You can order churnas, Ayurveda coffee, and other Ayurvedic foods from:

*Maharishi Ayur-Ved Products Intemat, Inc.
P.O. Box 49667
Colorado Springs, CO
80949-9667
Tel. 719-260-5500
and for orders
1-800-255-8332*

Braised Peppers with Spinach Rice
Pictured

• Bring a large pot of salted water to a boil. Rinse the rice in a colander. Rinse the spinach then place briefly in boiling water to blanch; refresh in cool water and chop fine. Heat ghee in another pan. Add bay leaf and coriander and heat until fragrant. Add rice and fry until it is translucent; add the spinach and fry together for about 1 minute. Carefully pour in ³/₄ cup boiling water, then cook over low heat for about 15 minutes.

• Meanwhile, wash and seed the peppers, then dice them fine. Heat 1 tablespoon ghee in a pan over medium heat; add fennel seeds and briefly sauté. Add bell peppers and sauté 1 minute. Add ¹/₄ cup plus 2 tablespoons water, salt, and black pepper; cook, covered, for about 10 minutes. To serve, mound rice in the center of a plate and place pepper mixture around it. Makes 2 servings.

Harmonize your dosha dominance:
Vata Very suitable without variations.
Pitta Use green bell peppers. Season with cream and turmeric. Sprinkle chopped herbs over top.
Kapha Braise the peppers in some water; add ghee at the end. In addition, season with ¹/₄ teaspoon each of ground ginger and ground coriander.

Cauliflower Curry
Classic

• Bring a large pot of salted water to a boil. Rinse the rice twice and let it drain in a colander; add the rice to the water, and let it simmer for about 15 minutes over low heat; drain and set aside, keeping warm.

• Meanwhile, clean and cut the cauliflower. Heat the ghee in a large pan, and add fennel, cumin, and anise seeds. Stir in turmeric. Add cauliflower and water; bring to a boil and let simmer, covered, for about 15 minutes. Stir in yogurt during the last 5 minutes of cooking time. Season with coriander, then serve with the rice. Makes 2 servings.

Harmonize your dosha dominance:
Vata Not suitable.
Pitta Don't use anise; add 1 teaspoon coriander, and serve with fresh herbs.
Kapha Don't use yogurt; add chili powder and freshly ground ginger. Use very little salt.

PER SERVING:		363 CALORIES
INFORMATION FOR PEPPER RECIPE		
Carbohydrate	44	g
Protein	5	g
Total fat	19	g
Cholesterol	49	mg
Sodium	175	mg
Fiber	5	g

PER SERVING:		222 CALORIES
INFORMATION FOR CURRY RECIPE		
Carbohydrate	29	g
Protein	6	g
Total fat	9	g
Cholesterol	26	mg
Sodium	190	mg
Fiber	2	g

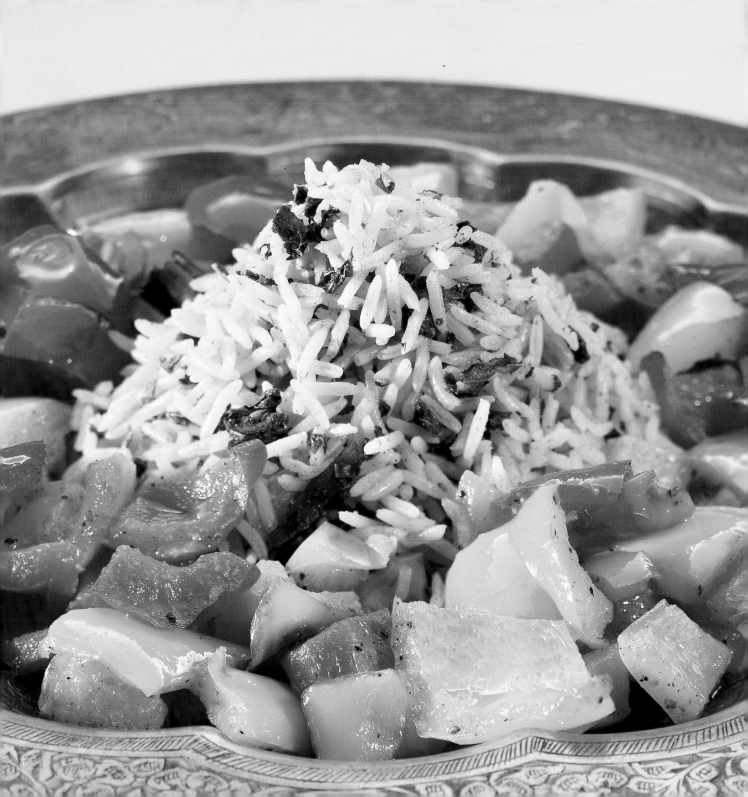

Vegetable Curry

2 carrots

1/3 lb (150 g) potatoes

1 (1-inch) piece fresh ginger

1/3 lb (150 g) fresh peas, shelled

1/2 teaspoon cumin seeds

1 teaspoon black mustard seeds (page 38)

1 teaspoon curry powder or churna (page 39)

freshly ground black pepper

1 tablespoon ghee

Preparation time: abut 50 minutes

Sweet Potatoes with Basil

1/2 teaspoon each: cumin seeds and coriander seeds

1 scant lb (400 g) sweet potatoes

1 tablespoon ghee

salt

freshly ground black pepper

5 sprigs basil

Preparation time: about 35 minutes

Vegetable Curry
Can be prepared in advance

• Peel the carrots and slice. Peel the potatoes and dice. Peel the ginger and slice thin. Combine peas, carrots, and potatoes in a large pot.

• Add ginger, cumin seeds, mustard seeds, and curry powder; add enough water to cover. Cover and cook over moderate heat for 20 to 25 minutes.

• Season with pepper, then stir in the ghee.

Harmonize your dosha dominance:
Vata If you can't get peas, use fresh green beans; season with 1/2 teaspoon thyme. Enrich with cream.
Pitta Don't use mustard seeds; add 1 teaspoon thyme or coriander. Enrich with cream.
Kapha Very suitable without any variations.

Sweet Potatoes with Basil
Pictured

• Grind cumin and coriander seeds in a spice grinder. Peel the sweet potatoes and slice.

• Heat the ghee in a large pan and add spices; briefly sauté spices over moderate heat. Add sweet potatoes and sauté. Add enough water to cover, and cook, covered, for about 15 minutes. Season with salt and pepper. Cut basil leaves into strips, and stir into the sweet potato mixture. Makes 2 servings.

Harmonize your dosha dominance:
Vata Leave out the coriander and substitute 1/4 teaspoon ground ginger.
Pitta Very suitable without variations.
Kapha Sweet potatoes are not suitable. Use bell peppers or all-purpose potatoes, and do not fry them but cook them in water. Add some ghee afterward; use less salt and season with ginger.

PER SERVING:	212 CALORIES
NUTRITIONAL INFORMATION	

Carbohydrate	34	g
Protein	6	g
Total fat	6	g
Cholesterol	16	mg
Sodium	31	mg
Fiber	9	g

PER SERVING:	293 CALORIES
NUTRITIONAL INFORMATION	

Carbohydrate	48	g
Protein	2	g
Total fat	11	g
Cholesterol	16	mg
Sodium	267	mg
Fiber	4	g

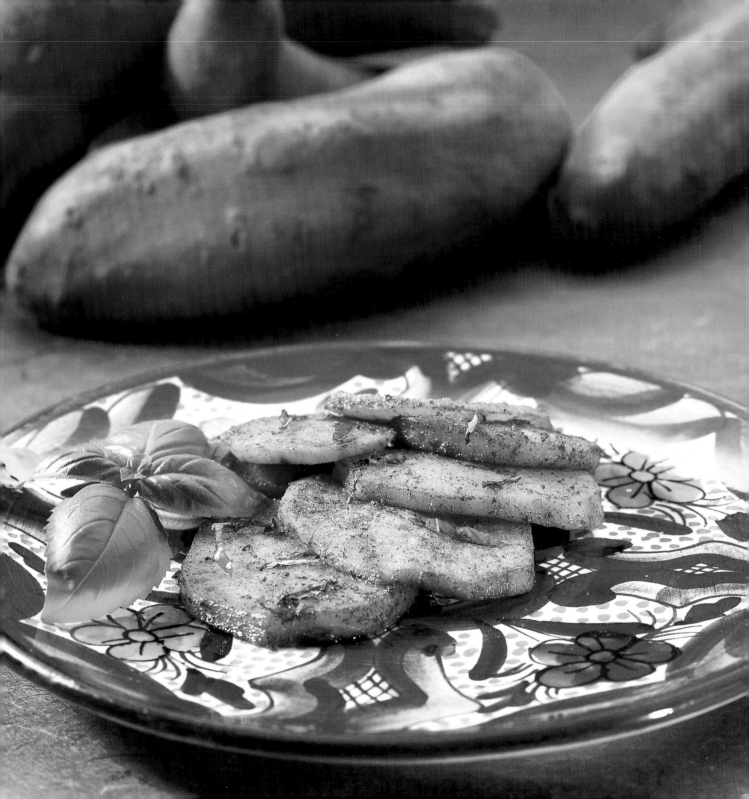

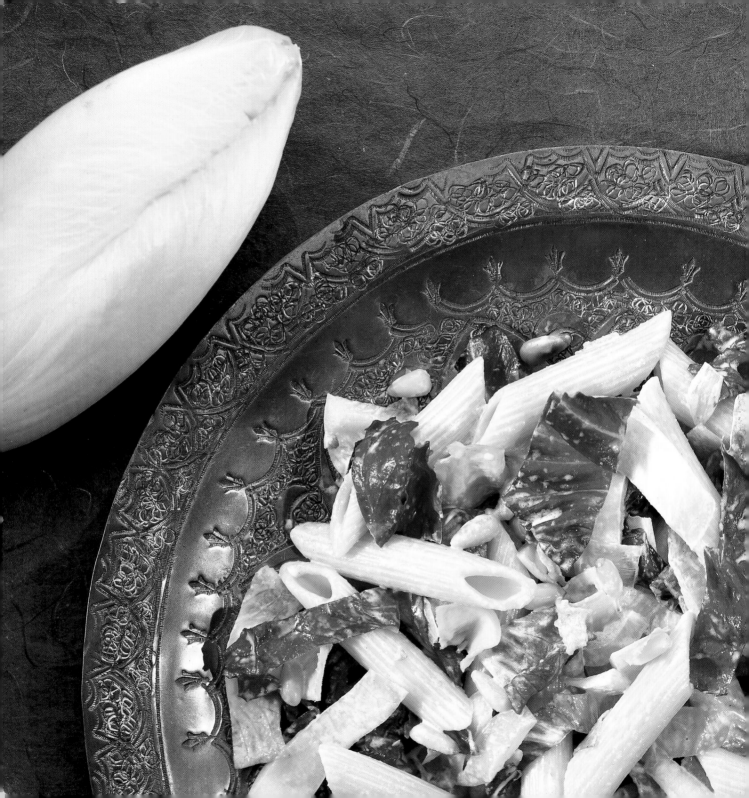

Radicchio and Vegetables with Penne
Best served very fresh

• Bring a large pot of salted water to a boil; add oil. Add pasta and let cook 10 minutes.

• In the meantime, halve the endive and radicchio heads, removing the stalk; cut leaves into strips. Seed the tomato and dice fine.

• Heat the ghee in a large pan. Grind coriander seeds in a spice grinder; add to pan and sauté over medium heat. Add the pine nuts and toast. Add the endive, radicchio, and tomato, and braise with a little water. Season with salt and pepper and cook, covered, over medium heat for about 5 minutes.

• Stir in the cream. Drain pasta, then mix with the vegetables. Makes 2 servings.

Harmonize your dosha dominance:
Vata Use cucumbers or zucchini instead of endive, radicchio, and tomato. Add dill or basil.
Pitta All pastas with cream sauces are especially well suited; you also may use more cream. In addition, use 1/2 teaspoon fennel seeds and some turmeric.
Kapha Use millet pasta. Instead of pine nuts, use sunflower seeds and 3 tomatoes. Braise the vegetables in water; add ghee at the end, leaving out the cream. Use salt sparingly.

Radicchio and Vegetables with Penne

salt
1 tablespoon sunflower oil
scant 1/2 lb (200 g) penne or spaghetti
1 head endive
1 small head radicchio
1 tomato
1 tablespoon ghee
1/2 teaspoon coriander seeds
2 tablespoons pine nuts
freshly ground black pepper
scant 1/2 cup (100 ml) cream

Preparation time: about 25 minutes

PER SERVING:	685 CALORIES	
NUTRITIONAL INFORMATION		
Carbohydrate 93	g
Protein 20	g
Total fat 27	g
Cholesterol 39	mg
Sodium 195	mg
Fiber 5	g

Asparagus with Sugar Snap Peas

sugar

²/₃ lb (300 g) asparagus

scant ¹/₄ lb (100 g) sugar snap peas

2 carrots

1 small zucchini

1 tablespoon ghee

¹/₂ teaspoon cumin seeds

scant ¹/₂ cup (100 ml) vegetable broth

2 tablespoons soy sauce

1 pinch freshly grated ginger

freshly ground black pepper

¹/₂ bunch chervil

Preparation time: about 50 minutes

Zucchini-Potato Cutlets

¹/₂ lb (250 g) potatoes

¹/₃ lb (150 g) zucchini

¹/₂ teaspoon each: coriander seeds and ground cumin

scant ¹/₂ cup (50 g) rolled oats

2 heaping tablespoons whole-wheat flour

salt

sweet paprika

freshly ground black pepper

3 tablespoons ghee

Preparation time: about 40 minutes

Asparagus with Sugar Snap Peas
Refreshing

• Bring a large pot of water to a boil with some sugar. Cut off the ends of the asparagus, and cut spears into pieces. Trim the pea pods and wash. Wash and peel the carrots, then slice thin. Halve the zucchini lengthwise, then slice. Cook the asparagus in the boiling water for 5 minutes, then drain.

• Heat ghee in a pan. Add cumin and sauté. Add the carrots and asparagus, and sauté briefly. Add the zucchini, pea pods, and broth, and cook, covered, for about 5 minutes. Season with soy sauce, ginger, and pepper. Sprinkle chervil leaves over top before serving. Makes 2 servings.

Harmonize your dosha dominance:
Vata Very suitable without variations.
Pitta In addition, add some coriander seeds with the cumin, and season with turmeric. Instead of soy sauce, use cream.
Kapha Cook vegetables in water with the spices and add ghee at the end. Spice it up with ginger.

PER SERVING:	228 CALORIES
NUTRITIONAL INFORMATION	
Carbohydrate 34	g
Protein 9	g
Total fat 7	g
Cholesterol 16	mg
Sodium .1159	mg
Fiber 6	g

Zucchini-Potato Cutlets
Pictured

• Peel and rinse the potatoes, then grate. Wash and trim the zucchini, then grate. Grind the coriander seeds fine in a spice grinder. In a large bowl, combine potatoes, zucchini, and coriander.

• Add cumin, rolled oats, and flour. Season with salt, paprika, and pepper; mix well.

• Heat ghee in a cast-iron pan. Form the vegetable mixture into six cutlets, then fry crispy-brown, turning once, over medium heat. Serve with hot cooked basmati rice and chutney. Makes 2 servings.

Harmonize your dosha dominance:
Vata Use carrots instead of zucchini. Instead of coriander, use ¹/₂ teaspoon fennel seeds and add ginger and nutmeg to taste.
Pitta Don't use any paprika. Also season with ¹/₄ teaspoon turmeric.
Kapha Anything fried or deep-fried is unsuitable. It's better to eat cooked vegetables with rice.

PER SERVING:	366 CALORIES
NUTRITIONAL INFORMATION	
Carbohydrate 43	g
Protein 7	g
Total fat 20	g
Cholesterol 49	mg
Sodium 154	mg
Fiber 5	g

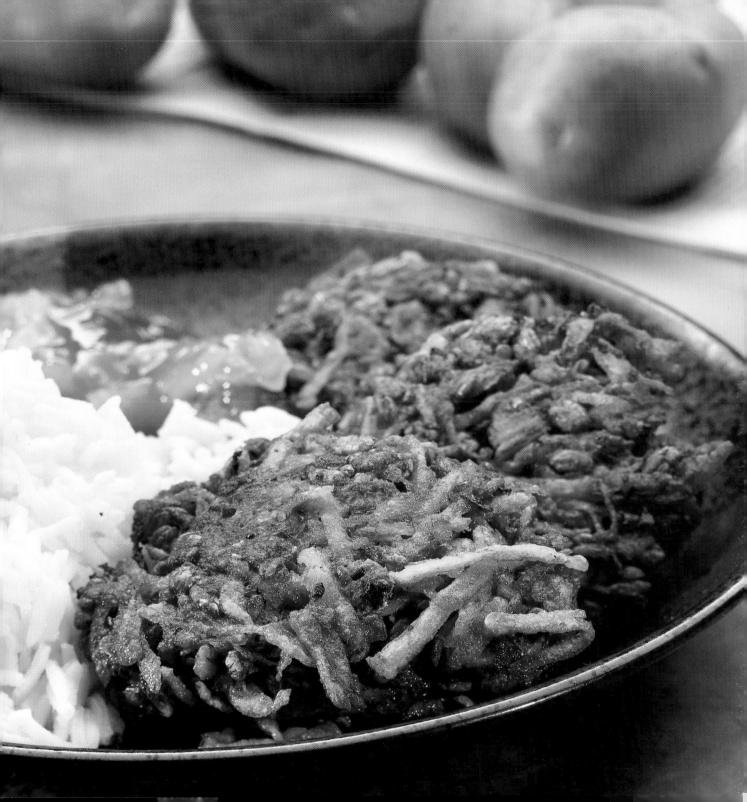

Potatoes with Curry Paste

²/₃ lb (300 g) potatoes

salt

1 (1-inch) piece fresh ginger

¹/₄ teaspoon each: turmeric
and fenugreek seeds
(page 39)

2 tablespoons ghee

1 teaspoon fennel seeds

Preparation time:
about 50 minutes

**Braised Beans and Corn
with Bulgur**

³/₄ cup plus 1¹/₂ tablespoons
(200 ml) vegetable broth

scant ¹/₄ lb (100 g) bulgur

¹/₂ teaspoon each: sweet
paprika and cumin seeds

¹/₄ teaspoon fenugreek seeds
(page 39)

generous ¹/₂ lb (250 g) green
beans

¹/₂ cup (150 g) frozen or
canned corn kernels, drained

1 tablespoon ghee

1 teaspoon black mustard
seeds (page 38)

grated peel of 1 lemon

salt

freshly ground black pepper

Preparation time:
about 1 hour

48

Potatoes with Curry Paste
Spicy

• Cook the potatoes, covered, in plenty of salted water for 20 minutes. Drain and let cool, then peel, and cut into small dice.

• Peel and grate the ginger. Grind turmeric, fenugreek, and 1 to 2 tablespoons water to a paste in a spice grinder.

• Heat the ghee in a frying pan. Add fennel seeds and sauté over medium heat. Add the spice paste and cook, stirring. Add potatoes, and sauté, stirring, for about 10 minutes, or until they are crispy-brown all over. Season with salt. Makes 2 servings.

Harmonize your dosha dominance:

Vata Use sweet potatoes instead of all-purpose potatoes. Cook, covered, 20 to 30 minutes, depending on their size.
Pitta Don't use fenugreek, but 1 teaspoon of thyme instead.
Kapha Kapha increases in food fried in ghee. Therefore you should instead use a spicy potato purée.

PER SERVING:	237 CALORIES	
NUTRITIONAL INFORMATION		
Carbohydrate	30	g
Protein	3	g
Total fat	12	g
Cholesterol	33	mg
Sodium	153	mg
Fiber	3	g

Braised Beans and Corn with Bulgur
Pictured

• Bring the broth to a boil in a medium-size saucepan. Add bulgur, paprika, and cumin. Let broth come to a boil again, then cook over low heat for about 20 minutes; set aside, keeping warm.

• Meanwhile, grind the fenugreek in a spice grinder. Heat the ghee in a large frying pan. Add mustard seeds and sauté until they start to jump. Add fenugreek and sauté briefly.

• Add beans, corn, and lemon peel, then cook, stirring, without browning. Season with salt and pepper, then add some water. Cover and cook over medium heat for about 20 minutes. Serve with the bulgur. Makes 2 servings.

Harmonize your dosha dominance:

Vata Very suitable without variations.
Pitta Prepare without paprika, mustard, and fenugreek seeds. Sauté with ¹/₂ teaspoon each of ground coriander, oregano, or basil.
Kapha Use millet instead of bulgur. Use less salt and season with ginger.

PER SERVING:	336 CALORIES	
NUTRITIONAL INFORMATION		
Carbohydrate	64	g
Protein	11	g
Total fat	7	g
Cholesterol	16	mg
Sodium	197	mg
Fiber	15	g

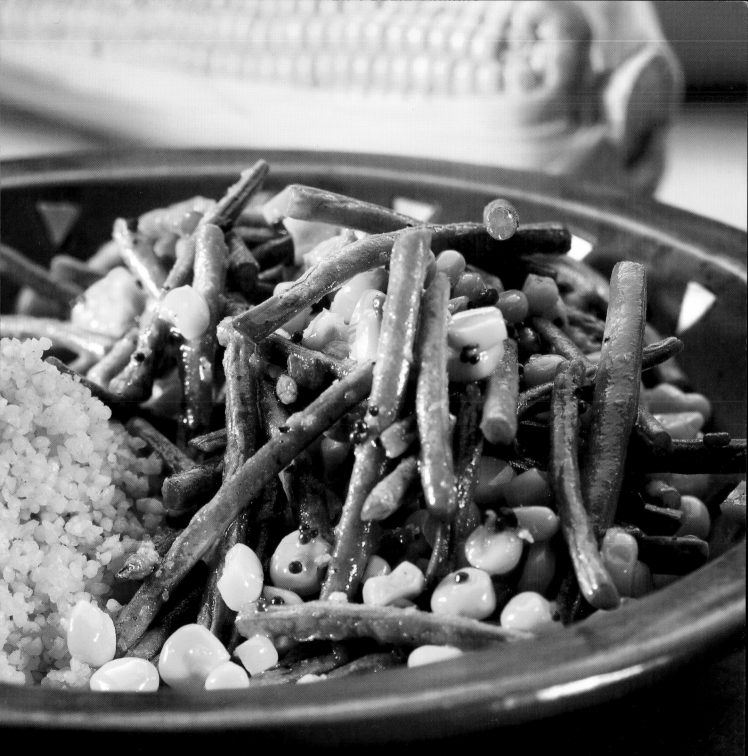

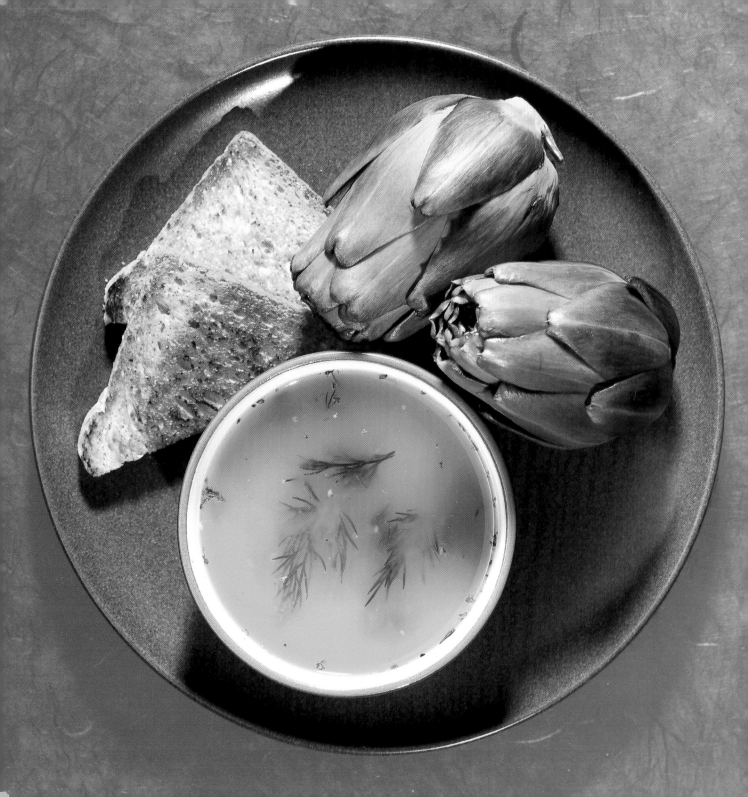

Artichokes with Herb Dip
Pictured

• Wash the artichokes and cut off the stems at the base. Bring a large pot of salted water to a boil; add 3 tablespoons lemon juice. Place artichokes in boiling water and let simmer for about 20 minutes, covered.

• Finely chop the herbs. In a small bowl, stir together 3 tablespoons lemon juice, pepper, salt, cayenne pepper, and gomashio. Beat in the oil and fold in the herbs. Serve whole artichokes with dipping sauce on the side.

• To eat, pull off the artichoke leaves one by one and dip them in the sauce. Eat with toasted whole-wheat bread. Makes 2 servings.

Harmonize your dosha dominance:
Vata Very suitable without variations.
Pitta For the dip, use cream instead of lemon juice, and leave out the cayenne.
Kapha Season the dip with ginger, and additional black pepper and cayenne.

Accompaniment for all doshas: curried rice
Cook a scant $1/2$ cup (100 g) basmati rice, then season with $1/2$ teaspoon turmeric, 1 teaspoon finely chopped fresh ginger, and 6 cardamom pods (or $1/2$ teaspoon cardamom seeds).

Cucumber Curry
Easy to prepare

• Peel the cucumber, quarter lengthwise, and scoop out the seeds. Cut the cucumber into slices.

• Bring the water to a boil with some salt. Rinse the rice, and cook in the boiling water for about 15 minutes.

• Grind the fennel seeds in a spice grinder. Add curry and some water, and work into a paste.

• Heat ghee in a pan. Add the paste and briefly sauté over medium heat. Add cucumber slices and cook, stirring. Stir in broth and cream, then cook, covered, for about 10 minutes. Season with pepper. Chop the dill and sprinkle over the curry before serving. Serve with the rice. Makes 2 servings.

Harmonize your dosha dominance:
Vata Very suitable without variations.
Pitta Very suitable without variations.
Kapha Not suitable.

PER SERVING:	252 CALORIES	
INFORMATION FOR ARTICHOKE RECIPE		
Carbohydrate	16	g
Protein	5	g
Total fat	21	g
Cholesterol	0	mg
Sodium	704	mg
Fiber	7	g

PER SERVING:	337 CALORIES	
INFORMATION FOR CURRY RECIPE		
Carbohydrate	46	g
Protein	6	g
Total fat	13	g
Cholesterol	39	mg
Sodium	197	mg
Fiber	2	g

Artichokes with Herb Dip

For the artichokes:
2 artichokes
salt
3 tablespoons fresh lemon juice

For the dip:
2 sprigs dill
$1/2$ bunch parsley
4 sprigs chervil
3 tablespoons fresh lemon juice
freshly ground black pepper
salt
1 pinch cayenne pepper
$1/2$ teaspoon gomashio (page 39)
3 tablespoons sunflower oil

Preparation time: about 30 minutes

Cucumber Curry

1 cucumber
$3/4$ cup (175 ml) water
salt
scant $1/2$ cup (100 g) basmati rice
$1/2$ teaspoon each: fennel seeds and curry powder or churna (page 39)
1 tablespoon ghee
scant $1/2$ cup (100 ml) vegetable broth
scant $1/2$ cup (100 ml) cream
freshly ground black pepper
1 small bunch of dill

Preparation time: about 30 minutes

51

Braised Okra with Basmati Rice

scant $1/2$ lb (200 g) carrots

scant $1/2$ lb (200 g) okra

$1/2$ red bell pepper

1 (1-inch) piece fresh ginger

$3/4$ cup (175 ml) water

salt

scant $1/2$ cup (100 g) basmati rice

5 black peppercorns

$1/4$ teaspoon fenugreek seeds (page 39)

2 tablespoons ghee

1 cup ($1/4$ l) vegetable broth

1 small cinnamon stick

$1/2$ bunch oregano

Preparation time: about 45 minutes

Bean-Coconut Curry

$2^{1}/2$ cups (600 ml) hot water

1 cup plus 2 tablespoons (125 g) flaked coconut

scant $1/2$ lb (200 g) carrots

scant $1/2$ lb (200 g) haricots verts

1 tablespoon ghee

churna (page 39)

salt

freshly ground black pepper

Preparation time: about 45 minutes

Braised Okra with Basmati Rice
Classic

• Wash and trim the carrots, then slice diagonally. Trim okra and cut in half horizontally. Cut bell pepper into diamond shapes. Peel and grate the ginger.

• Bring the water to a boil with salt. Rinse the rice, then cook in the water for 15 minutes.

• Meanwhile, crush the peppercorns and fenugreek. Heat the ghee in a large frying pan. Add spices and briefly sauté over medium heat. Add ginger and briefly sauté. Add the vegetables, and heat through without browning, stirring constantly; pour in the broth. Add the cinnamon stick and oregano leaves, then cook, covered, for about 10 minutes. Serve with rice. Makes 2 servings.

Harmonize your dosha dominance:
Vata In addition, use $1/2$ teaspoon black mustard seeds and churna.

Pitta Use green bell pepper. In addition, season with $1/2$ teaspoon coriander and some turmeric.

Kapha Cook the vegetables, with the spices, in the vegetable broth, and stir in the ghee at the end.

PER SERVING:	336 CALORIES	
NUTRITIONAL INFORMATION		
Carbohydrate	66	g
Protein	7	g
Total fat	5	g
Cholesterol	11	mg
Sodium	240	mg
Fiber	6	g

Bean-Coconut Curry
Pictured

• In a medium-size bowl, combine the hot water and coconut; let soak. Trim the vegetables. Peel the carrots, and slice thin; halve the beans if necessary.

• Heat the ghee in a large pan. Add the spices and sauté briefly; add the vegetables and cook, stirring. Season with salt and pepper. Place a fine-meshed strainer over the pan; pour coconut-water mixture into the strainer. Pressing with your hand, squeeze all the water into the pan. Cook the curry, covered, in the coconut water over low heat for about 20 minutes. Serve with hot-cooked rice. Makes 2 servings.

Harmonize your dosha dominance:
Vata For the spices, sauté $1/4$ teaspoon cumin seeds, ginger, some ground fenugreek, $1/2$ teaspoon chopped basil or oregano, and 1 pinch of asafetida.

Pitta For the spices, use $1/2$ teaspoon ground coriander, $1/2$ teaspoon fennel seeds, ginger, cumin seeds, and turmeric. Prepare without carrots.

Kapha For the spices, add $1/2$ teaspoon each of ginger, ground coriander, and turmeric to the coconut water. Add some ghee at the end.

PER SERVING:	457 CALORIES	
NUTRITIONAL INFORMATION		
Carbohydrate	52	g
Protein	8	g
Total fat	27	g
Cholesterol	16	mg
Sodium	392	mg
Fiber	11	g

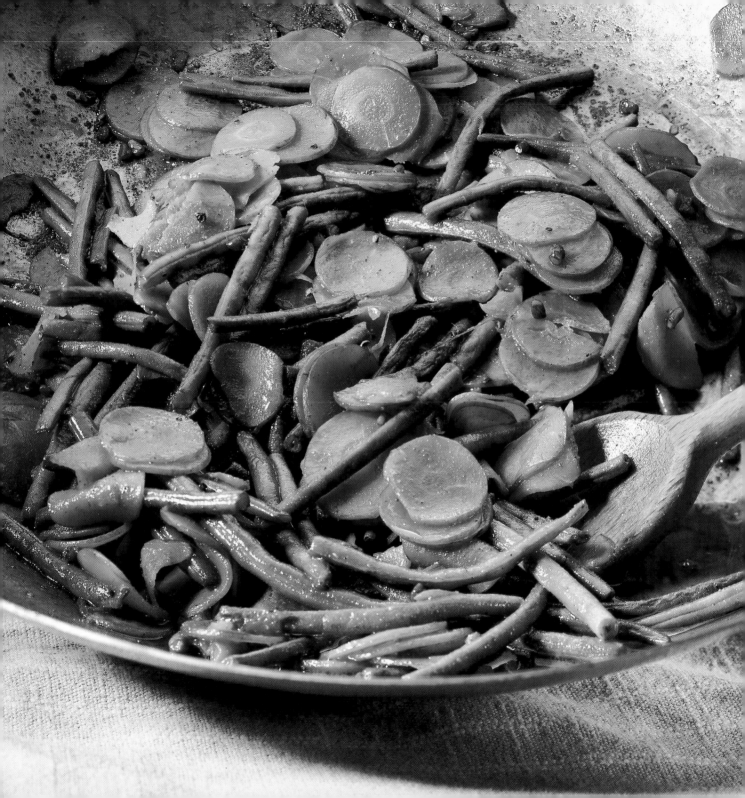

Small, round, strong!

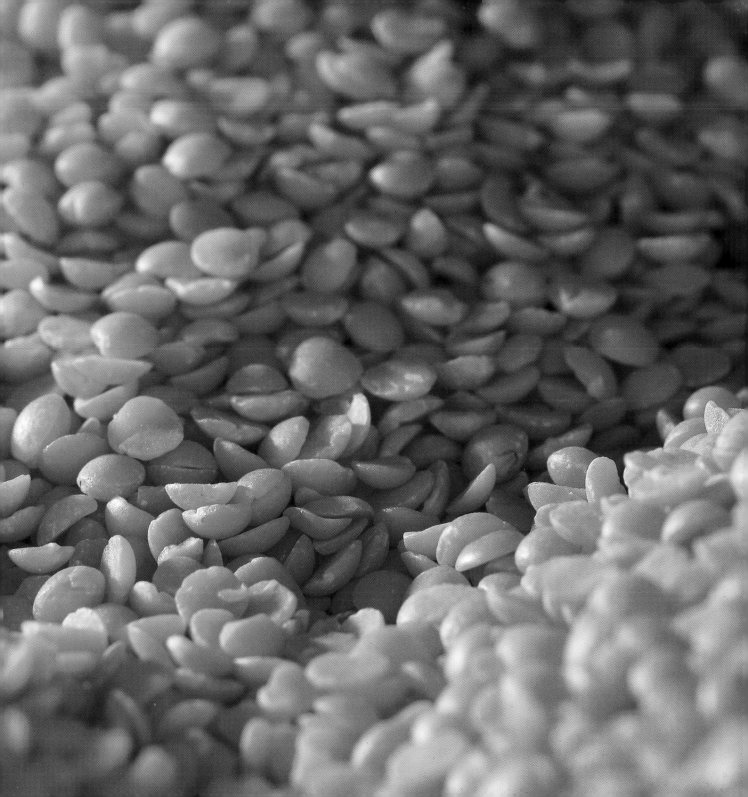

Grains and Dal

Dal has two forms: split lentils and peas are called *dal*—and dal also is the name for the souplike dish that is prepared from them. A small serving of dal should be offered regularly at the main meal; it contains valuable vegetable protein, as well as iron and B complex vitamins. There are more than fifty varieties of dal, the most common of which we introduce to you here. Dal is available in Middle Eastern and Indian food stores and some grocery stores.

• Mung dal—from the mung bean, can be green or yellow, which is made from hulled beans. Mung dal is used frequently and has a mild flavor. Properly prepared, it is easily digestible and is suitable for small children.

• Chickpeas—are available just about everywhere. The peas have a unique shape and are light brown. When dried, they are very hard and should be softened overnight before being cooked.

• Chickpea flour—also known as besan or gram flour, is a pale yellow flour made from ground, dried chickpeas. It can be found in Indian and Asian markets. Store, wrapped airtight, in the refrigerator for up to six months.

• Channa dal—a small relative of the chickpea, has a yellowish color. Its flavor is slightly sweet. If you can't get channa dal use yellow mung dal or yellow split peas.

• Red lentils—are quite well known. They cook very fast and do not need to be softened.

Preparation of dal

In preparing dal, it is important to soften it well and cook it long enough. Dal must be fully cooked so that it takes on a creamy consistency. Cook dal in a large pot, because, as it boils, a foam develops, which should be skimmed off from time to time. Add the spices after the dal stops foaming—or add the seared spices at the end. It is important to stir the dal well so that it doesn't burn.

In general all legumes easily stimulate Vata and can cause gas. Therefore the dal should not only be well cooked, but also well seasoned. That way, you can reduce the Vata-increasing effect. Asafetida is often used to season dal, and it prevents the formation of gas by breaking down indigestible enzymes.

Dal is recommended for any dosha dominance. But it is very suitable for Kapha dominance, since legumes primarily have a tart taste.

Grains, or cereal grains, also are important in the Ayurvedic diet. They are a readily available source of protein and have more carbohydrates than any other food. Some of the more popular grains include barley, bulgur, corn, millet, oats, quinoa, rice, and rye.

Bulgur—is wheat kernels that have been steamed, dried, and crushed; it is not the same as cracked wheat. Bulgur has a nutty flavor and tender, chewy texture.

Millet—has a bland flavor that lends itself well to seasonings.

Quinoa—has a delicate flavor that has been compared to couscous. This tiny bead-shaped grain is considered a complete protein because it contains all eight essential amino acids. Quinoa cooks like rice, taking half the time of regular rice, and expands to four times its original volume.

The Taste Lines: Six Rasas

We recognize six different taste lines or rasas: sweet, sour, salty, hot, bitter, and tart.

Vata is soothed and balanced with sweet, sour, salty.

Pitta is soothed and balanced with sweet, bitter, and tart.

Kapha is soothed and balanced with hot, bitter, and tart.

Examples for the six rasas:

Sweet: Rice, bread, milk, butter, ghee, oils, sugar, fruit that is ripe and sweet

Sour: Lemon, tomatoes, yogurt

Salty: Salt

Hot: Hot spices, such as pepper, ginger, paprika, curry powder

Bitter: All vegetables and lettuces

Tart: Legumes, honey, rhubarb, cabbage

All six rasas should be present in one meal, or at least be eaten during the course of a day. Give preference to the taste lines that balance your dosha dominance, but include the other rasas in your food as well.

Note: None of our recipes contain garlic or onions. Garlic has a long list of medicinal effects and is very stimulating. According to the Maharishi Ayurveda, garlic and onions are not used in cooking because they influence the sense of taste.

Cooking for Several People—the Tastes Are Different

Would you like to cook type-specific food for several people? Place all the food separately on the table—salads, vegetables, rice—and let each person take what and how much he wants.

The recipe suggestions don't mean that you may eat only *according to your dosha dominance; the quantity also is critical. Give preference to the foods for your dosha dominance.*

Prepare the dishes in such a way that they can be altered individually. This means that each person should add his own salt, cream, ghee, or lemon, according to his own taste. Spices also can be added later.

A simple way to make the dishes fit different tastes, is to season them with churnas (page 39).

Wheat Curry

1/3 lb (150 g) wheat grains

1 1/2 cups (350 ml) vegetable broth

2 ribs celery

2 tablespoons ghee

1/2 teaspoon anise seeds

2 teaspoons churna or curry powder (page 39)

1/2 cup (75 ml) cream

salt

sambal oelek (see page 39)

Preparation time: about 1 1/4 hours (+ overnight soaking)

Yellow Mung Dal

scant 1/4 cup (100 g) yellow mung dal

1 heaping teaspoon freshly grated ginger

1 pinch ground fenugreek (page 39)

1/2 teaspoon each: cumin and black onion seeds (pages 38–39)

1 teaspoon each: turmeric and fennel seeds

1 bay leaf

2 cloves

1 teaspoon ground coriander

salt

1 pinch ground asafetida (page 38)

Preparation time: 45–60 minutes (+ overnight soaking)

58

Wheat Curry
Spicy

• Soften the wheat in a large pot of water overnight. Let drain in a sieve. Bring vegetable broth to a boil in a large saucepan. Add the wheat and cook, covered, for about 50 minutes over low heat; drain and set aside.

• Trim and wash the celery, then slice. Heat the ghee in a pan. Finely grind the anise in a spice grinder. Add anise and churna to the ghee and sauté over moderate heat. Add celery and sauté briefly. Add wheat to the pan; sauté, but do not brown. Add some water and the cream. Season with churna, salt, and sambal oelek, then cook, covered, for about 15 minutes. Makes 2 servings.

Harmonize your dosha dominance:
Vata and **Pitta** Don't use sambal oelek; the curry could be too hot for you.
Kapha Don't braise the celery, but cook it in water with the spices and a little salt. Don't use cream.

PER SERVING:	480 CALORIES
NUTRITIONAL INFORMATION	
Carbohydrate 68	g
Protein 13	g
Total fat 20	g
Cholesterol 55	mg
Sodium 792	mg
Fiber 7	g

Yellow Mung Dal
Pictured

• Wash and pick over the mung dal. Place in a large bowl with enough water to cover; soak 15 minutes. Drain the mung dal in a sieve. Place mung dal and 1 1/4 cups (300 ml) water in a large saucepan; bring to a boil, skimming the foam. Add the spices and cook, uncovered, over medium heat for 20 to 30 minutes or until the dal begins to cook down. Stir well during cooking, adding water if necessary. Season with salt and asafetida. Makes 2 servings.

Well suited for all doshas:
Eat it regularly! Well cooked and seasoned, it is easily digested.

Variations:
Herb dal (pictured)
Stir in parsley, cilantro, and dill.

Southern Indian dal
Add palm sugar, flaked coconut, and cream.

Dal soup
Dal can occasionally be warmed up. Warm the leftovers, add more water as needed, then season some more and it's done!

PER SERVING:	168 CALORIES
NUTRITIONAL INFORMATION	
Carbohydrate 32	g
Protein 10	g
Total fat 3	g
Cholesterol 0	mg
Sodium 162	mg
Fiber 8	g

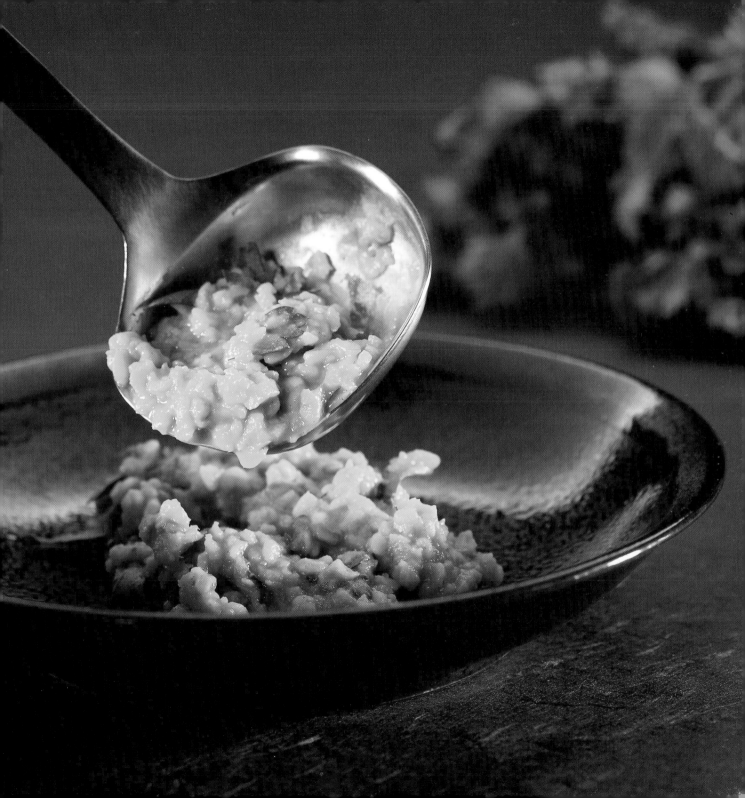

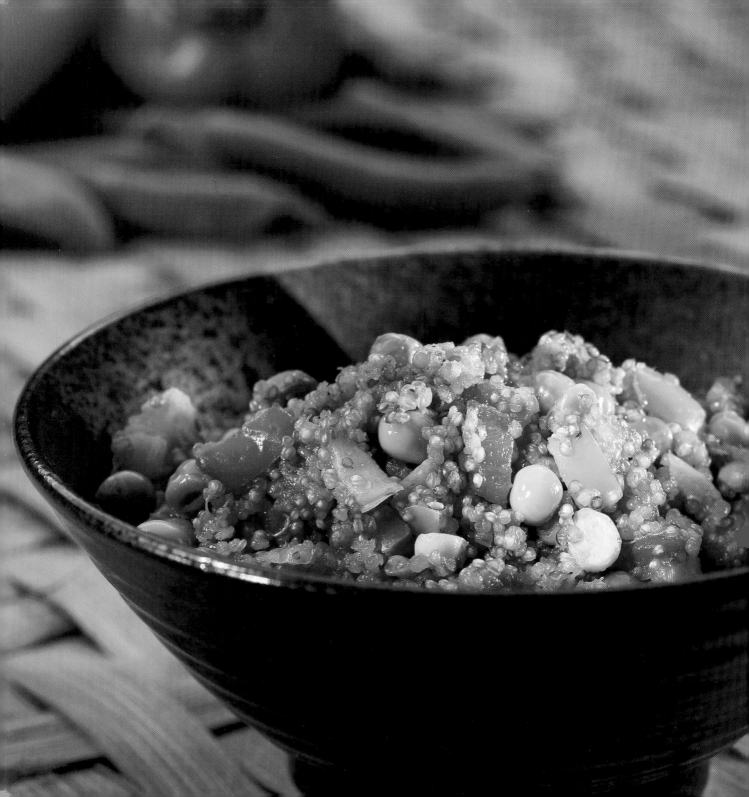

Green Spelt Soufflé
More time-consuming

• Rinse the green spelt and let it drain. In a large saucepan, combine spelt, water, paprika, curry, and salt. Bring to a boil, then cook, covered, over low heat for about 25 minutes. Drain in a sieve.

• Meanwhile, preheat the oven to 350° F (175° C). Grease an 8-inch-square baking dish with ghee. Drain the tomatoes, reserving the juice. In a small bowl, combine juice with cream. Finely chop the tomatoes. Combine tomatoes, cream mixture, spelt, and thyme leaves in the baking dish. Bake in the oven for about 45 minutes. Makes 2 servings.

Harmonize your dosha dominance:
Vata Very suitable without variations.
Pitta Tomatoes are not suitable for Pitta dominance; only use a little, preferably without seeds, which will lessen the acidity. Leave out the paprika and season with turmeric and Pitta churna.
Kapha More suitable grain varieties are barley, millet, or buckwheat. In addition, use 1 to 2 teaspoons freshly ground ginger.

PER SERVING:	267 CALORIES	
NUTRITIONAL INFORMATION		
Carbohydrate 23		g
Protein 9		g
Total fat 14		g
Cholesterol 45		mg
Sodium 1094		mg
Fiber 5		g

Quinoa Risotto with Peas
Pictured

• Shell the peas. Clean, wash, and dice the peppers. Heat the ghee in a pan. Add quinoa and briefly sauté over medium heat.

• Add the peas, bell peppers, broth and lemon juice, then cook, covered, over medium heat for about 20 minutes. Season with salt, black pepper, and paprika. Makes 2 servings.

Harmonize your dosha dominance:
Vata Use basmati rice instead of spelt. In addition, sauté ¹/₂ teaspoon cumin seeds in the ghee.
Pitta Use little lemon juice, no paprika, and green bell peppers instead of red. Use additional herbs, such as marjoram, basil, thyme, as well as ¹/₂ teaspoon ground coriander, and some turmeric for seasoning.
Kapha Use buckwheat instead of spelt. In addition, season with ginger and cumin. Use little salt.

PER SERVING:	564 CALORIES	
NUTRITIONAL INFORMATION		
Carbohydrate 88		g
Protein 21		g
Total fat 16		g
Cholesterol 33		mg
Sodium 216		mg
Fiber 20		g

Green Spelt Soufflé
¹/₄ lb (125 g) green spelt
1 cup (¹/₄ l) water
¹/₂ teaspoon sweet paprika
¹/₄ teaspoon curry powder or churna (page 39)
salt
1 (28 oz/800 g) can peeled tomatoes
1 scant cup (200 ml) cream
1 bunch lemon thyme

For the baking dish:
ghee

Preparation time:
about 1 hour 20 minutes
(45 minutes of which is baking time)

Quinoa Risotto with Peas
1 scant lb (400 g) fresh peas
¹/₂ each: red and yellow bell peppers
2 tablespoons ghee
¹/₄ lb (125 g) quinoa (page 57)
1 cup (¹/₄ l) vegetable broth
2 tablespoons fresh lemon juice
salt
freshly ground black pepper
sweet paprika

Preparation time:
about 40 minutes

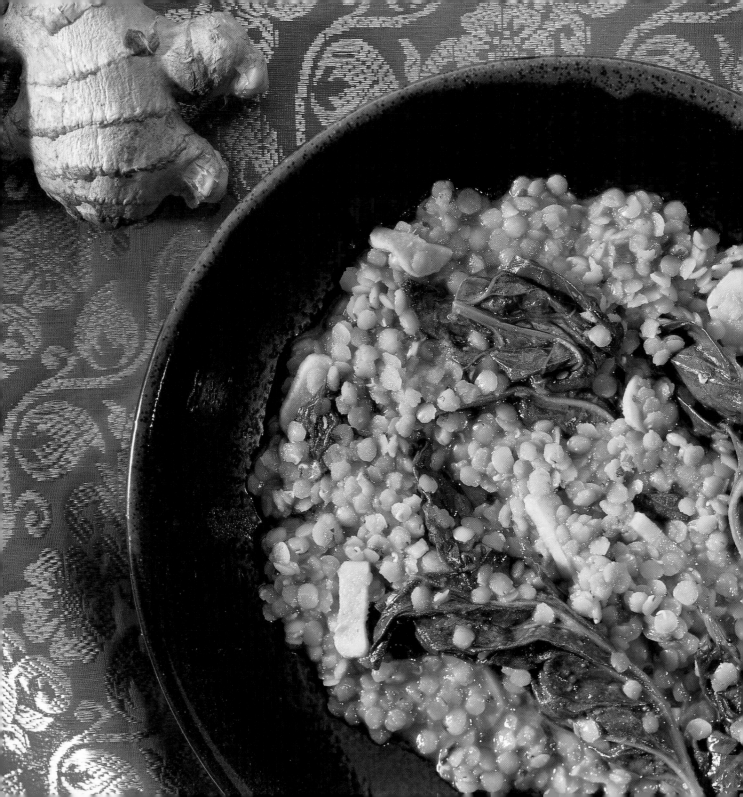

Red Lentils with Ginger
Pictured

• In a large saucepan, bring the broth and paprika to a boil. Rinse the lentils twice, let drain, then add to the broth and let simmer for about 20 minutes.

• Meanwhile, wash and pick over the spinach. Peel the ginger and cut into thin slices. Heat ghee in a large pan. Add cumin and ginger and sauté briefly. Add wet spinach leaves, and steam, covered, for about 10 minutes.

• Drain the lentils, then add to the spinach. Finely chop the cilantro, and stir into lentil mixture. Season with lemon juice, sugar, and pepper. Makes 2 servings.

Harmonize your dosha dominance:
Vata Very suitable without variations.
Pitta Instead of lentils, use yellow mung dal. Let dal soften overnight, then cook for about 20 minutes without paprika. Don't use lemon, but flavor with cream.
Kapha Don't sauté the spices. Cook the spinach and spices in water, then season according to taste.

PER SERVING:		297 CALORIES
NUTRITIONAL INFORMATION		
Carbohydrate 42	g
Protein 20	g
Total fat 7	g
Cholesterol 16	mg
Sodium 147	mg
Fiber 20	g

Chickpeas with Tomatoes
Suitable for guests

• Soften chickpeas overnight in a large bowl of water to cover.

• Let chickpeas drain in a sieve. In a large saucepan, combine chickpeas, broth, bay leaf, and fennel seeds. Bring to a boil, then cook, covered, over low heat for about 45 minutes, or until the chickpeas are soft.

• Peel and grate the ginger. Halve the tomatoes, remove the stem and seeds, then dice coarsely.

• Heat ghee in a pan. Add the tomatoes, ginger, and asafetida, then cook, without browning, over medium heat. Add the drained chickpeas, and let cook, covered, for about 10 minutes. Season with salt and pepper. Chop cilantro and stir in. Makes 2 servings.

Harmonize your dosha dominance:
Vata Very suitable without variation.
Pitta Use 1 tomato.
Kapha Very suitable without variations. Use little salt.

PER SERVING:		260 CALORIES
NUTRITIONAL INFORMATION		
Carbohydrate 32	g
Protein 8	g
Total fat 12	g
Cholesterol 16	mg
Sodium 425	mg
Fiber 7	g

Red Lentils with Ginger
1 scant cup (200 ml) vegetable broth
1/2 teaspoon sweet paprika
scant 1/4 lb (100 g) red lentils
scant 1/2 lb (200 g) spinach leaves
1 (1-inch) piece fresh ginger
1 tablespoon ghee
1/2 teaspoon cumin seeds
1 bunch cilantro
fresh lemon juice to taste
1 pinch sugar (preferably palm sugar)
freshly ground black pepper

Preparation time: about 30 minutes

Chickpeas with Tomatoes
scant 1/4 lb (75 g) chickpeas
1 scant cup (200 ml) vegetable broth
1 bay leaf
1/2 teaspoon fennel seeds
1 (1-inch) piece fresh ginger
3 to 4 tomatoes
1 pinch ground asafetida
1 tablespoon ghee
salt
freshly ground black pepper
1/2 bunch cilantro

Preparation time: about 1 hour (+ overnight soaking)

63

Yellow Mung Dal with Vegetables

scant $^1/_4$ cup (50 g) mung beans
2 carrots
scant $^1/_2$ lb (200 g) fresh peas
2 cups ($^1/_2$ l) hot water
1 tablespoon ghee
$^1/_2$ teaspoon fennel seeds
1 teaspoon freshly grated ginger
$^1/_2$ teaspoon cumin seeds
1 teaspoon turmeric
1 pinch ground asafetida (page 38)
fresh lemon juice to taste
salt
$^1/_2$ teaspoon granulated sugar

Preparation time:
about 1 hour
(+ overnight soaking)

Coconut Dal

scant $^1/_4$ cup (50 g) channa dal (page 56)
1 bay leaf
1 small cinnamon stick
4 cardamon pods
2 cups ($^1/_2$ l) water
1 tablespoon ghee
$^1/_2$ teaspoon cumin seeds
$^1/_4$ teaspoon anise seeds
$^1/_2$ teaspoon ground ginger
1 teaspoon turmeric
1 pinch ground asafetida (page 38)
2 tablespoons flaked coconut
2 tablespoons granulated sugar
scant $^1/_2$ cup (100 ml) cream
salt

Preparation time:
45 to 60 minutes
(+ 4 hours soaking time)

Yellow Mung Dal with Vegetables
Pictured

• Rinse the mung beans, then place in a large bowl with enough water to cover; soften overnight.

• Wash and trim the carrots, then slice thin. Shell and wash the peas.

• Drain the mung beans in a sieve. Combine mung beans and water in a large saucepan and bring to a boil. Cook about 20 minutes over medium heat, skimming the foam from time to time. Add the carrots and peas, then cook for 10 to 15 minutes more.

• Heat the ghee in a pan. Add spices and sauté briefly; stir spice mixture into the dal. Season with lemon juice, salt, and sugar. Makes 2 servings.

Harmonize your dosha dominance:
Vata Very suitable without variations.
Pitta Don't use lemon juice; flavor with cream.
Kapha Don't use sugar, and use only a little salt; add cayenne pepper.

Coconut Dal
Classic

• Soften the channa dal in a large pot of water to cover, for about 4 hours; drain in a sieve. Combine the dal, bay leaf, cinnamon stick, cardamom pods, and water in a large pot and bring to a boil. Cook over medium heat for 30 to 45 minutes, frequently skimming off the foam. Stir occasionally.

• Heat the ghee in a pan. Add the cumin and anise, and sauté briefly, stirring; add remaining spices and sauté briefly. Add coconut and continue to sauté, stirring. Stir the ghee-spice mixture, sugar, and cream into the dal, then let simmer for about 10 minutes more. Season with salt. Makes 2 servings.

Harmonize your dosha dominance:
Vata Very suitable without variations.
Pitta Very suitable without variations.
Kapha Leave out the cream. Spice it up with ginger, black pepper, and Kapha churna.

PER SERVING:	273 CALORIES	
NUTRITIONAL INFORMATION		
Carbohydrate 42	g
Protein 13	g
Total fat 7	g
Cholesterol 16	mg
Sodium 274	mg
Fiber 13	g

PER SERVING:	287 CALORIES	
NUTRITIONAL INFORMATION		
Carbohydrate 33	g
Protein 8	g
Total fat 15	g
Cholesterol 39	mg
Sodium 184	mg
Fiber 4	g

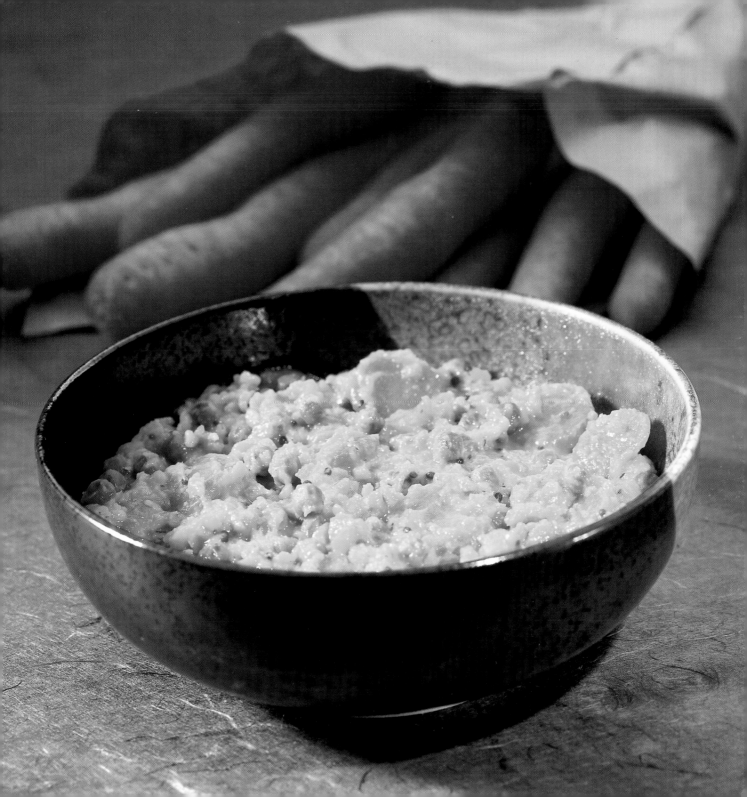

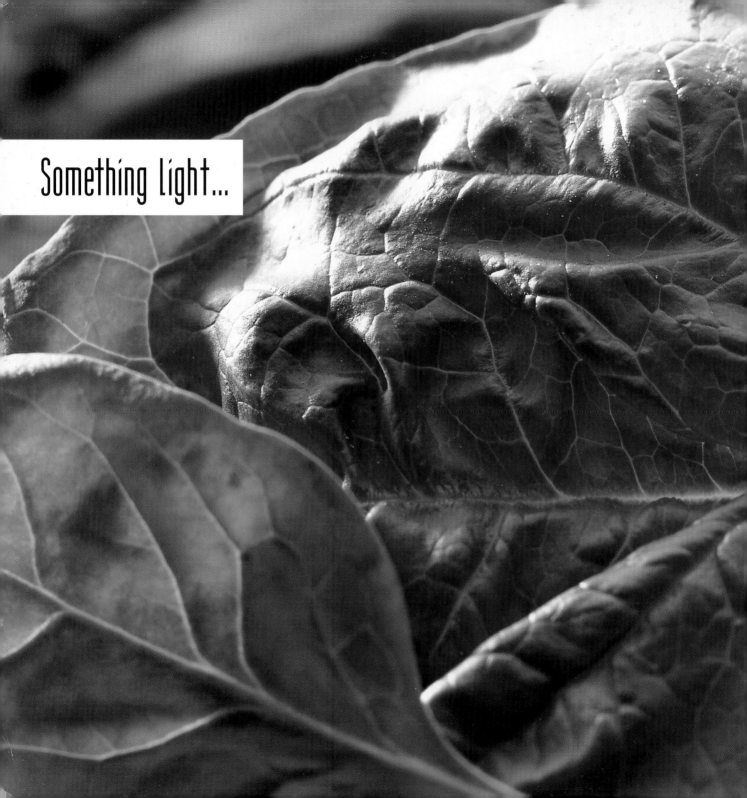

Something light...

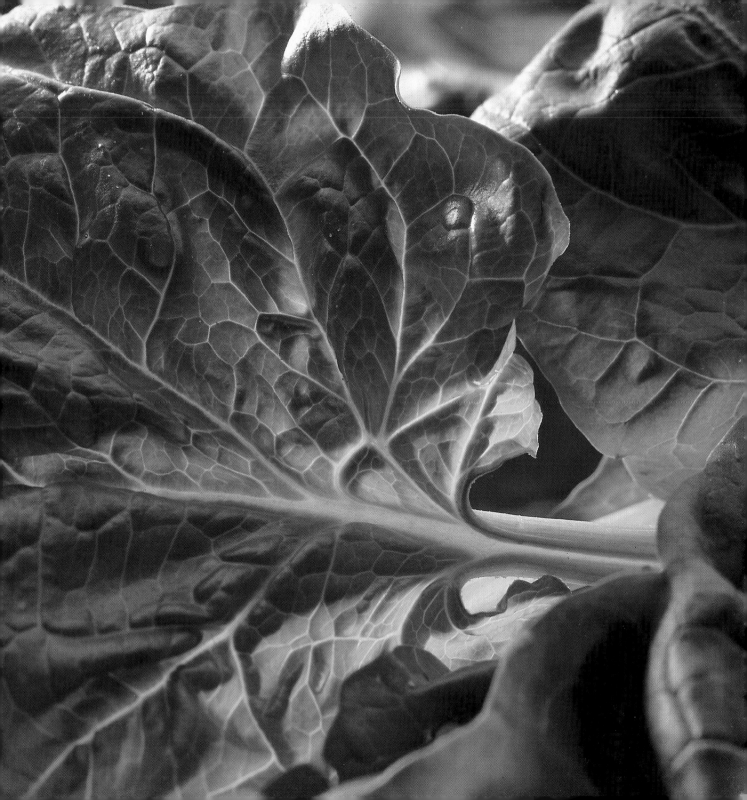

Soups and Stews

The dishes in this chapter are very suitable for light evening meals. Read our Ayurvedic recommendations for the evening meal on page 69.

Diet in Harmony with the Cosmos

In the Ayurveda, we start with the premise that many influences affect us. Everything is connected to everything else and influences us reciprocally. We also are constantly exposed to change, for example, the seasons, changing climates, different times of day, and the different phases of life (see front cover flap). Our working conditions and our moods change, as well. All these factors have an influence on our doshas, which means that the dosha dominance can change over the short term or long term. Perhaps the Pitta or fire element is so strongly stimulated in you during the summer, or by a heated discussion, that ice cream is exactly the right cooler. However, if you have a Vata dominance, ice cream is not necessarily considered beneficial.

You should constantly pay attention to what your body tells you, and practice self-awareness. The Ayurveda offers guidelines that you can use to personalize your diet. You should prepare food not only according to your dosha dominance and season, but also to your taste and what is easily digestible.

Breakfast

If you aren't hungry in the morning, some fruit, a glass of milk, or freshly squeezed fruit juice may be enough for you.

Some people aren't hungry until after 10 A.M., when the Pitta period begins. What you eat during that time is digested better than in the preceding Kapha period. Have a cup of spiced or herb tea with toast or a roll, honey, or fresh cheese—depending on your taste and dosha dominance. In fall and winter, hot cereal with raisins and nuts is very satisfying.

The Midday Meal

The midday meal should be the main meal of the day, because the digestive power is at its greatest around noon the high point of the Pitta period (see front cover flap).

The Evening Meal

For supper, the Ayurveda recommends light food. If possible, eat by 6 P.M., when the Kapha period begins, and the body begins to slow down. If you eat later than 6 P.M., the food should be even lighter. Since the liver works according to certain rhythms, you should eat hot food and avoid such proteins as meat, fish, sausage, and cheese or soy products. You also should avoid sour milk products in the evening.

So, what can you eat in the evening? Soups, pasta dishes with cream sauces, and vegetables on toast are ideal for the Kapha period. You are only limited to your imagination. The food doesn't need to be fancy or take a long time to prepare.

Free of Waste Products (Ama)

When you eat light foods in the evening, you relieve your body and will wake up fresher the next morning. Meal proteins are difficult to metabolize at night. Sitting in the stomach, the incomplete digestion produces metabolic waste products called ama.

The body tries to protect itself from these waste products, or poisons, by storing them in the small capillaries or tissues. There, the ama collects over time, and can lead to illness and disease. Thus, the Ayurveda considers the diet an important form of disease prevention. These metabolic processes make it vital that you eat only when you are hungry. The previous meal should be completely digested before you eat again. If you already eat only when you are hungry, then just eat warm light soups and drink plenty of warm water (see page 85).

Purifying the Body

It is best to undertake a regular purification, at least once a year. This means to follow a special diet for ama reduction, and to undergo a panchakarma cure—an intensive Ayurvedic cleansing procedure. This consists of oil massages and other natural procedures. Write to the address listed on page 39 for more information.

Jerusalem Artichoke Cream

1/2 lb (250 g) sunchokes
salt
1/2 teaspoon fennel seeds
1 tablespoon ghee
1 cup (1/4 l) water
1 scant cup (200 ml) cream
freshly ground black pepper
fresh lemon juice

Preparation time:
about 40 minutes

Asparagus Soup

3 carrots
1 2/3 lb (750 g) asparagus
1 head kohlrabi
1 tablespoon ghee
1 cup plus 1 tablespoon
(250 ml) vegetable broth
salt
freshly ground black pepper
1/4 teaspoon ground coriander
1 slice whole-wheat bread
1 tablespoon wheat germ oil
3 sprigs chervil

Preparation time:
about 45 minutes

Jerusalem Artichoke Cream
Pictured

• Clean sunchokes under running water. Bring a large pot of salted water to a boil; add sunchokes and cook for 8 to 10 minutes. Drain sunchokes, then peel and chop; set aside.

• Grind the fennel seeds fine in a spice grinder. Heat the ghee in a large frying pan. Add the fennel seeds and sauté over moderate heat.

• Add sunchokes and sauté about 3 minutes. Pour in the water and cream, then season with black pepper. Let simmer, covered, for about 15 minutes. Cool several minutes, then purée in the food processor and stir in lemon juice before serving. Makes 2 servings.

Harmonize your dosha dominance:
Vata Season with nutmeg and ginger. Serve with chopped cilantro sprinkled overtop.
Pitta Don't use any lemon juice. Serve with a lot of chopped parsley.
Kapha Cook the sunchokes and spices in 2 cups (1/2 l) water. Season with ginger, ground black pepper, and paprika. Only use a dash of cream.

PER SERVING:	299 CALORIES	
NUTRITIONAL INFORMATION		
Carbohydrate	26	g
Protein	6	g
Total fat	20	g
Cholesterol	61	mg
Sodium	200	mg
Fiber	2	g

Asparagus Soup
A new way to prepare a classic

• Wash and peel the carrots; thinly slice. Cut off the tough ends of the asparagus, then cut the spears into pieces. Peel the kohlrabi and chop small.

• Heat the ghee in a large pot. Add vegetables and cook without browning. Pour in the broth, then season with salt, pepper, and coriander, and cook, covered, for about 20 minutes.

• Meanwhile, toast the bread in a pan without any fat. Remove from pan and brush with oil. Pull chervil leaves off the stems, and sprinkle leaves on the bread. Divide soup between 2 bowls. Cut the chervil toast in half diagonally, and garnish each bowl with a half.

Harmonize your dosha dominance:
Vata Leave out the kohlrabi and coriander. Season at the end with Vata churna.
Pitta Use potatoes instead of carrots. Season at the end with Pitta churna.
Kapha Cook the vegetables in broth instead of fat. Season with ginger, and Kapha churna, using little salt.

PER SERVING:	277 CALORIES	
NUTRITIONAL INFORMATION		
Carbohydrate	32	g
Protein	14	g
Total fat	11	g
Cholesterol	16	mg
Sodium	361	mg
Fiber	11	g

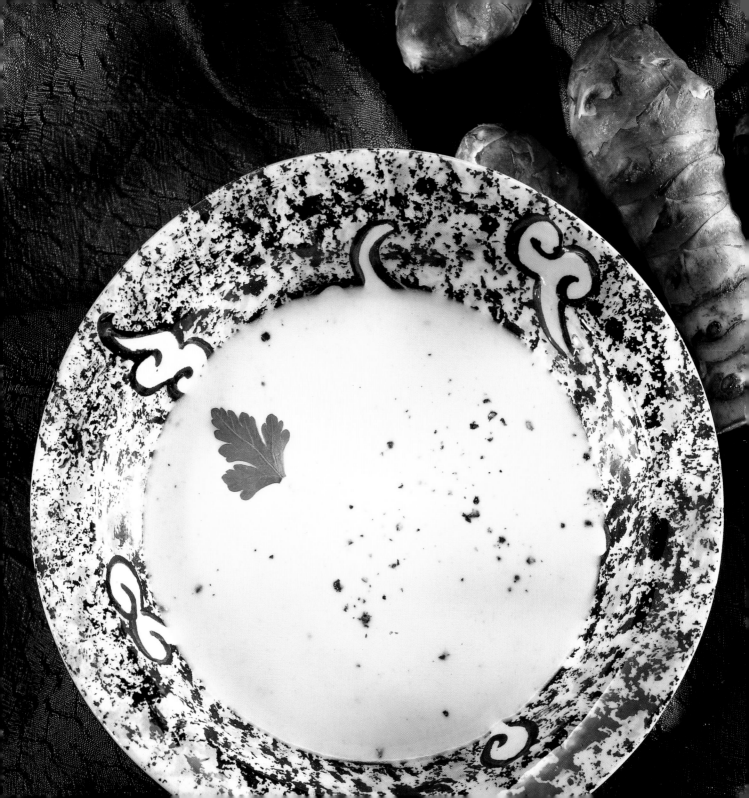

Broccoli Soup with Mint

2/3 lb (300 g) broccoli
1 (1-inch) piece fresh ginger
1/4 teaspoon cumin seeds
1/2 teaspoon coriander seeds
1 tablespoon ghee
1 1/2 cup plus 2 tablespoons (375 ml) vegetable broth
2 sprigs mint
scant 1/2 cup (100 ml) cream
salt
freshly ground black pepper

Preparation time: about 45 minutes

Lentil Curry Soup

1/4 lb (100 g) potatoes
1/2 teaspoon cumin seeds
1 teaspoon coriander seeds
1 tablespoon ghee
1 teaspoon turmeric
1 tablespoon curry powder or churna (page 39)
scant 1/4 cup (50 g) red lentils
2 cups (1/2 l) vegetable broth
salt
freshly ground black pepper
fresh lemon juice
cilantro leaves

Preparation time: about 1 hour

Broccoli Soup with Mint
Pictured

• Clean the broccoli and cut into florets; peel and slice the stems. Peel and grate the ginger.

• Grind cumin and coriander seeds in a spice grinder. Heat the ghee in a pot. Add the ground spices and briefly sauté; add broccoli, and continue cooking without browning. Pour in the vegetable broth. Add the ginger and mint sprigs, then bring to a boil and let simmer, covered, for about 20 minutes.

• Remove the mint and purée the soup. Return the soup to the pot, and stir in the cream; bring to a boil, then season with salt and black pepper. Makes 2 servings.

Harmonize your dosha dominance:
Vata Use carrots instead of broccoli, and simmer with 3 bay leaves. Use 1 teaspoon fennel seeds instead of coriander.
Pitta Very suitable without variations.
Kapha Don't sear the spices. Cook broccoli and spices in the broth. Add the ghee at the end. Use less cream. Season with Kapha churna, using little salt.

PER SERVING:	204 CALORIES
NUTRITIONAL INFORMATION	
Carbohydrate . . . . .17 g	
Protein . . . . .7 g	
Total fat . . . . .14 g	
Cholesterol . . . . .39 mg	
Sodium .281 mg	
Fiber . . . . .4 g	

Lentil Curry Soup
Suitable for guests

• Peel and dice the potatoes. Grind the cumin and coriander seeds in a spice grinder.

• Heat ghee in a pot. Add ground spices, turmeric, and curry, and sauté over medium heat. Add the potatoes and lentils and cook without browning. Pour in the broth and bring to a boil. Let simmer, covered, for about 35 minutes. Purée, then season with salt, pepper, and lemon juice. Garnish with cilantro leaves.

Harmonize your dosha dominance:
Vata Use fennel seeds instead of coriander. Cook with 2 whole cloves, removing them before puréeing. Season with nutmeg and caraway.
Pitta Use softened mung dal; use 1 teaspoon fennel seeds instead of cumin. Season with cream rather than lemon juice.
Kapha Cook in 1 to 2 teaspoons freshly grated ginger and 2 whole cloves.

PER SERVING:	226 CALORIES
NUTRITIONAL INFORMATION	
Carbohydrate . . . . .35 g	
Protein . . . . .9 g	
Total fat . . . . .6 g	
Cholesterol . . . . .16 mg	
Sodium .246 mg	
Fiber . . . . .8 g	

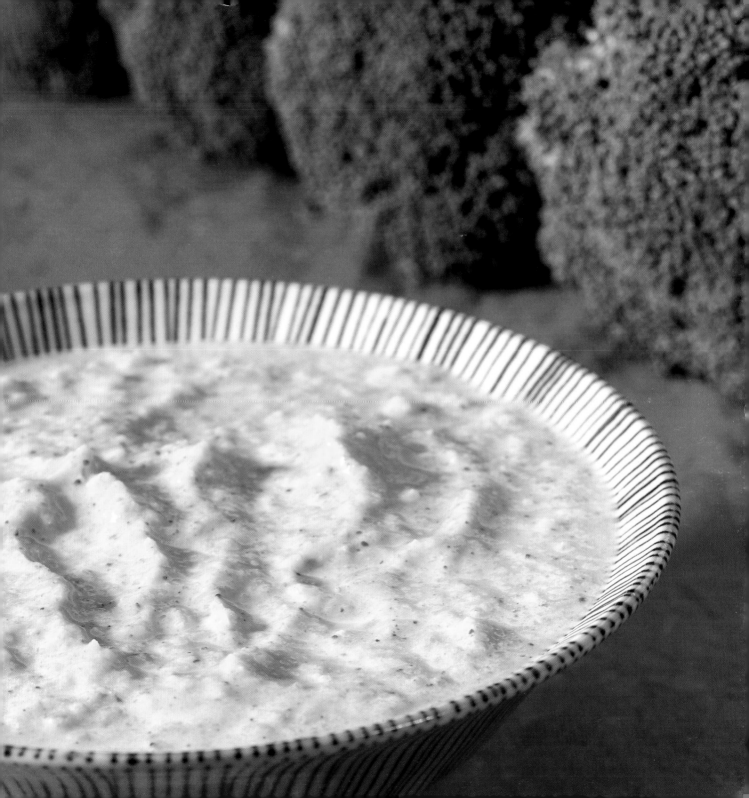

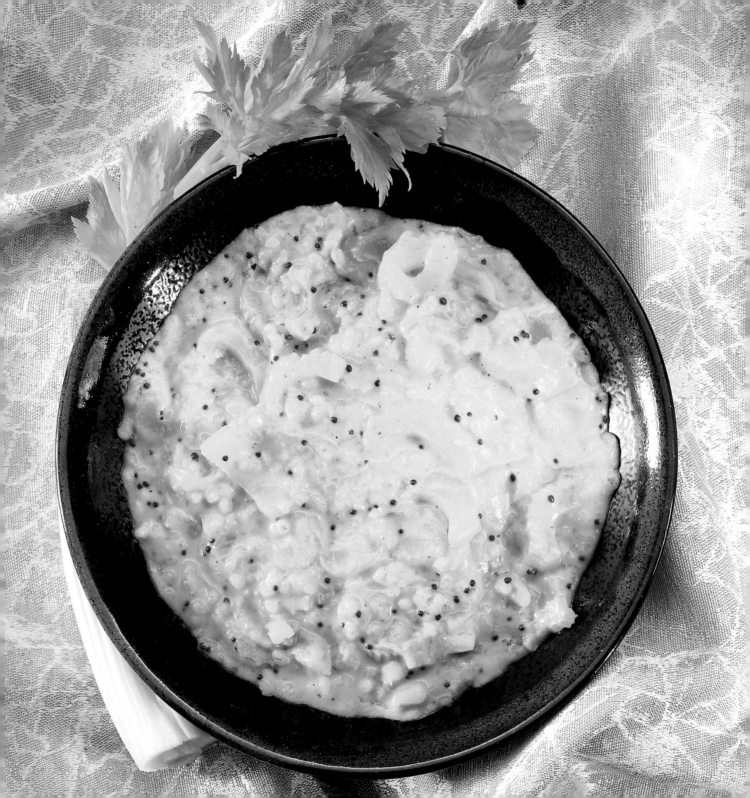

Cucumber Soup
Easy to prepare

• Peel the cucumber; split it lengthwise, scoop out the seeds with a spoon, and dice small. Finely chop the dill.

• Combine the broth and cucumber in a large pot. Bring to a boil, then add the cream. Place mixture in a food processor and purée. Stir in the dill, then season with salt and pepper; set aside.

• Grind the fennel seeds fine in a spice grinder. Heat the ghee in a small pan, and add the fennel; sauté briefly.

• Serve the soup lukewarm in soup bowls and top with the fennel seeds and ghee. Makes 2 servings.

Harmonize your dosha dominance:
Vata Suitable without variations.
Pitta Suitable without variations.
Kapha Not suitable.

Curry Soup with Pearl Barley
Pictured

• Trim the celery and cut into slices. Grind the coriander seeds in a spice grinder. Heat the oil in a pot. Add mustard seeds, and sauté over medium heat. Add the celery and coriander, then heat without browning.

• Sprinkle the curry and flour in the pan, and cook, stirring. Pour in the broth. Add the barley, bring to a boil, and cook for about 10 minutes over medium heat. Stir in the cream, then season with salt and pepper. Makes 2 servings.

Harmonize your dosha dominance:
Vata Depending on your tastes, sauté ¹/₂ teaspoon fennel seeds with the mustard seeds. Instead of barley, stir cooked rice into the soup.
Pitta Instead of mustard seeds, use ¹/₂ teaspoon turmeric.
Kapha Prepare without flour, salt, and cream. Cook the celery in broth without heating it in the ghee. Add 1 teaspoon freshly grated ginger.

Cucumber Soup
1 small cucumber
¹/₂ bunch dill
1 cup (¹/₄ l) vegetable broth
¹/₂ cup plus 2 tablespoons (150 ml) cream
salt
freshly ground black pepper
1 teaspoon fennel seeds
1 tablespoon ghee

Preparation time: about 25 minutes

Curry Soup with Pearl Barley
1 rib celery
¹/₂ teaspoon coriander seeds
1 tablespoon sunflower oil
¹/₂ teaspoon mustard seeds
1 tablespoon curry powder or churna (page 39)
1 tablespoon whole-wheat flour
2 cups (¹/₂ l) vegetable broth
¹/₄ cup (50 g) pearl barley
scant ¹/₄ cup (50 ml) cream
salt
freshly ground black pepper

Preparation time: about 25 minutes

PER SERVING:	197 CALORIES	
NUTRITIONAL INFORMATION		
Carbohydrate	13	g
Protein	4	g
Total fat	15	g
Cholesterol	44	mg
Sodium	239	mg
Fiber	1	g

PER SERVING:	183 CALORIES	
NUTRITIONAL INFORMATION		
Carbohydrate	33	g
Protein	5	g
Total fat	4	g
Cholesterol	11	mg
Sodium	273	mg
Fiber	5	g

Savoy Cabbage Soup

1 1/8 lb (500 g) savoy cabbage
1 carrot
1/4 teaspoon anise seeds
2 cups (1/2 l) vegetable broth
scant 1/4 cup (50 g) red lentils
2 whole cloves
freshly ground black pepper
ground ginger
turmeric

Preparation time:
about 50 minutes

Herb Soup

1 tablespoon ghee
1 teaspoon curry powder or
churna (page 39)
1 teaspoon whole-wheat
flour
2 cups (1/2 l) vegetable broth
scant 1/2 cup (100 ml) cream
1 bunch parsley
5 sprigs lemon balm
2 sprigs mint
3 sprigs cilantro
1/2 bunch tarragon
salt
freshly ground black pepper

Preparation time:
about 20 minutes

Savoy Cabbage Soup
Pictured

• Clean the cabbage and cut into strips. Peel and slice the carrot.

• Grind the anise in a spice grinder. In a large pot, combine the broth, lentils, carrots, cabbage, and cloves; bring to a boil, and let simmer for about 20 minutes over medium heat. Season with pepper, ginger, and turmeric.

Harmonize your dosha dominance:
Vata Not suitable.
Pitta Instead of the carrot, use 1 medium-size (150 g) potato and no red lentils. Season with cream.
Kapha Very suitable without variations.

Tip:
The quality of the ingredients are very important in this simple soup. If possible, use organic savoy cabbage; it won't have the typical cabbage smell. The soup should smell very good.

PER SERVING:	206 CALORIES
NUTRITIONAL INFORMATION	
Carbohydrate 42	g
Protein 13	g
Total fat 6	g
Cholesterol 0	mg
Sodium 181	mg
Fiber 16	g

Herb Soup
Easy to prepare

• Heat the ghee in a large pot. Sprinkle in the curry and flour, then brown. Pour in the broth and cream and let cook for about 10 minutes over medium heat.

• Remove the leaves from the herb sprigs; chop the leaves, and add to the soup. Purée the soup in a food processor, then season with salt and pepper.

Harmonize your dosha dominance:
Vata Instead of parsley, use 3 to 4 sprigs basil.
Pitta Instead of lemon balm, use a lot of dill.
Kapha Browned flour is not suitable. Instead, serve the hot vegetable broth without the flour and ghee mixture. Season with ginger and Kapha churna.

PER SERVING:	191 CALORIES
NUTRITIONAL INFORMATION	
Carbohydrate 14	g
Protein 4	g
Total fat 13	g
Cholesterol 39	mg
Sodium 286	mg
Fiber 1	g

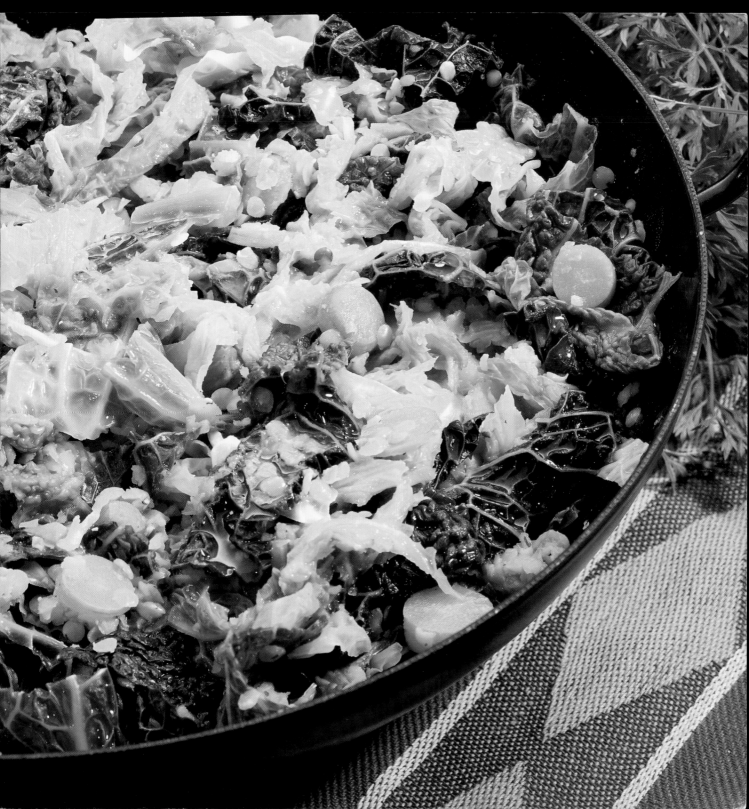

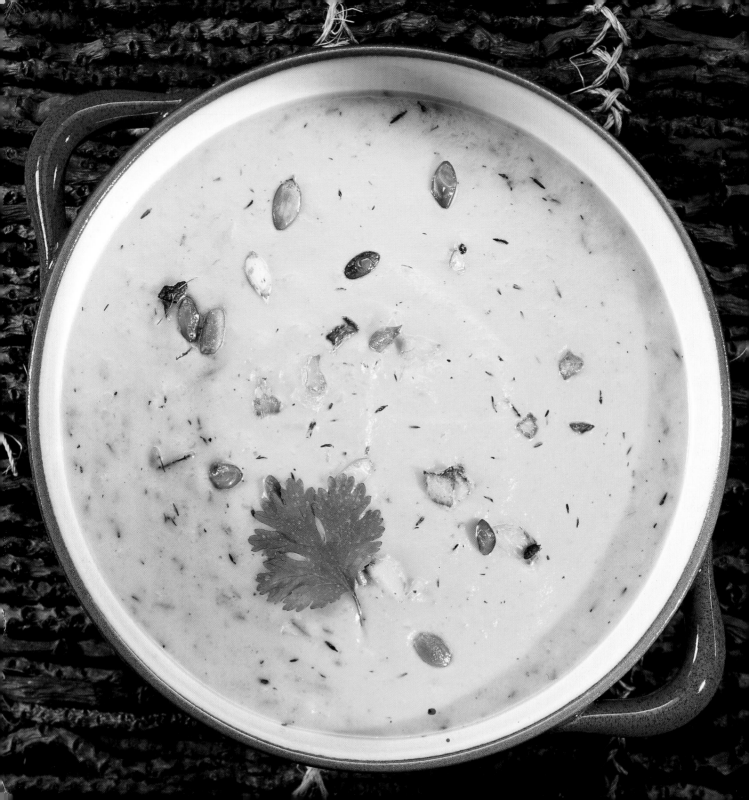

Pumpkin Soup
Pictured

• Peel and dice the pumpkin. Peel and dice the potato.

• Heat ghee in a large pot over medium heat. Grind the rosemary in a spice grinder, then sauté briefly in ghee. Add potato and sauté briefly, then add pumpkin and sauté again. Pour in the broth and bring to a boil. Season with salt and pepper, then let simmer, covered, for about 25 minutes, stirring frequently.

• Purée the soup in a food processor, then stir in the cream; set aside.

• Peel the ginger and slice very thin. Heat the oil in a small pan and add ginger and pumpkin seeds; sauté until aromatic. Divide soup between 2 bowls, then top with pumpkin seeds, ginger, and cilantro. Makes 2 servings.

Harmonize your dosha dominance:
Vata Well suited without variations.
Pitta Well suited without variations.
Kapha Prepare without cream, using little salt. Don't sauté spices in oil and ghee; cook all in the broth. Season with hot spices.

PER SERVING:	421 CALORIES	
NUTRITIONAL INFORMATION		
Carbohydrate 41	g
Protein 11	g
Total fat 26	g
Cholesterol .39	mg
Sodium .330	mg
Fiber 8	g

Green Spelt Soup with Spinach
Very nutritious

• Rinse the spelt twice. Heat the ghee in a large pot. Add spelt, paprika, and coriander and sauté over medium heat. Add the broth, and pepper, then bring to a boil. Simmer, covered, for about 30 minutes.

• Meanwhile wash and pick over the spinach, then finely chop. Remove basil leaves from the stems.

• Add the spinach and cream to the soup, then cook for 5 minutes more. Stir in the basil and serve with toast. Makes 2 servings.

Harmonize your dosha dominance:
Vata Sauté 1/4 teaspoon fennel seeds with paprika.
Pitta Season without using paprika; use coriander and some turmeric instead.
Kapha Instead of green spelt use barley. Don't sear the herbs. Add ginger to season. Cook without cream.

PER SERVING:	446 CALORIES	
NUTRITIONAL INFORMATION		
Carbohydrate 62	g
Protein 15	g
Total fat 17	g
Cholesterol .44	mg
Sodium .287	mg
Fiber 5	g

Pumpkin Soup
1 1/8 lb (500 g) pumpkin
1 medium-size (150 g) potato
1 tablespoon ghee
1/2 teaspoon rosemary
1 1/2 cups (350 ml) vegetable broth
salt
freshly ground black pepper
scant 1/2 cup (100 ml) cream
1 (1-inch) piece fresh ginger
2 tablespoons pumpkin seeds
1 tablespoon oil
cilantro leaves

Preparation time: about 1 hour

Green Spelt Soup with Spinach
1/4 lb (100 g) green spelt
1 tablespoon ghee
1/2 teaspoon sweet paprika
1/4 teaspoon ground coriander
2 cups (1/2 l) vegetable broth
freshly ground black pepper
1/2 lb (200 g) spinach leaves
10 basil leaves
1/2 cup plus 2 tablespoons (150 ml) cream
1 slice whole-wheat toast

Preparation time: about 45 minutes

Vegetable Stew

1 beet
about $^1/_2$ lb (200 g) potatoes
2 carrots
about $^1/_2$ lb (200 g) white cabbage
1 bay leaf
2 cups ($^1/_2$ l) vegetable broth
freshly ground black pepper
ground ginger
2 teaspoons ghee

Preparation time:
about 1 hour

Cauliflower Soup

1 small head cauliflower
1 (1-inch) piece fresh ginger
1 tablespoon ghee
$^1/_2$ teaspoon black mustard seeds (page 38)
$1^3/_4$ cups (400 ml) vegetable broth
scant $^1/_2$ cup (100 ml) cream
salt
freshly ground black pepper

Preparation time:
about 40 minutes

Vegetable Stew
Pictured

• Peel the beet under running water, then dice. Peel and dice the potatoes. Peel and slice the carrots. Clean the cabbage and cut into strips.

• In a large pot, combine the vegetables, broth, and bay leaf, and bring to a boil; let boil covered, for about 30 minutes, over moderate heat. Season with pepper and ginger. Stir in the ghee before serving. Remove bay leaf. Makes 2 servings.

Harmonize your dosha dominance:
Vata Don't use cabbage; use more carrots. In addition, season with thyme, nutmeg, and fennel, or add Vata churna.
Pitta Instead of carrots and beets, use green beans and peas. Season lightly. In addition, use basil or oregano, turmeric, and cream for seasoning.
Kapha Very suitable without variations. Season with Kapha churna, if desired.

Cauliflower Soup
Spicy

• Clean the cauliflower and cut into florets. Peel the ginger and chop fine.

• Heat the ghee in a pot. Add the mustard seeds and sauté over medium heat until they start to jump (be careful not to let them burn). Add the ginger and cauliflower, and cook without browning. Pour in the broth; bring quickly to a boil, then cook, covered, for about 15 minutes. Remove from heat and stir in the cream; season with salt and pepper. Makes 2 servings.

Harmonize your dosha dominance:
Vata Cauliflower is not suitable; use beets. Sauté $^1/_2$ teaspoon cumin seeds with mustard seeds.
Pitta Sauté $^1/_2$ teaspoon coriander seeds with mustard seeds; season with turmeric.
Kapha Don't use cream; add little salt. Sauté $^1/_2$ teaspoon each of cumin seeds and coriander seeds with the mustard seeds. Season with nutmeg, or ground cloves and turmeric.

PER SERVING:	246 CALORIES
NUTRITIONAL INFORMATION	
Carbohydrate 48	g
Protein 6	g
Total fat 5	g
Cholesterol 11	mg
Sodium 173	mg
Fiber 7	g

PER SERVING:	182 CALORIES
NUTRITIONAL INFORMATION	
Carbohydrate 13	g
Protein 4	g
Total fat 13	g
Cholesterol 39	mg
Sodium 263	mg
Fiber 2	g

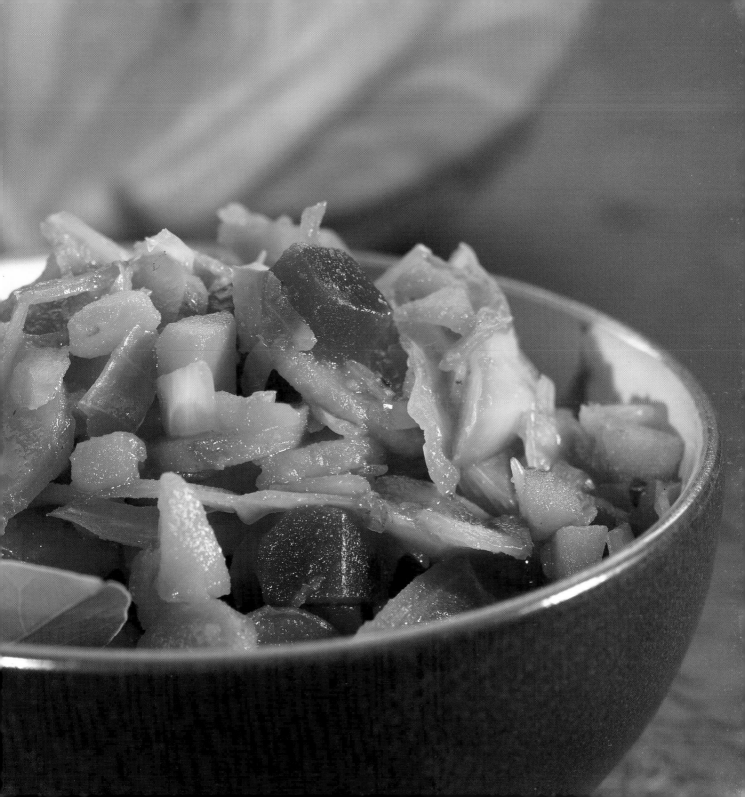

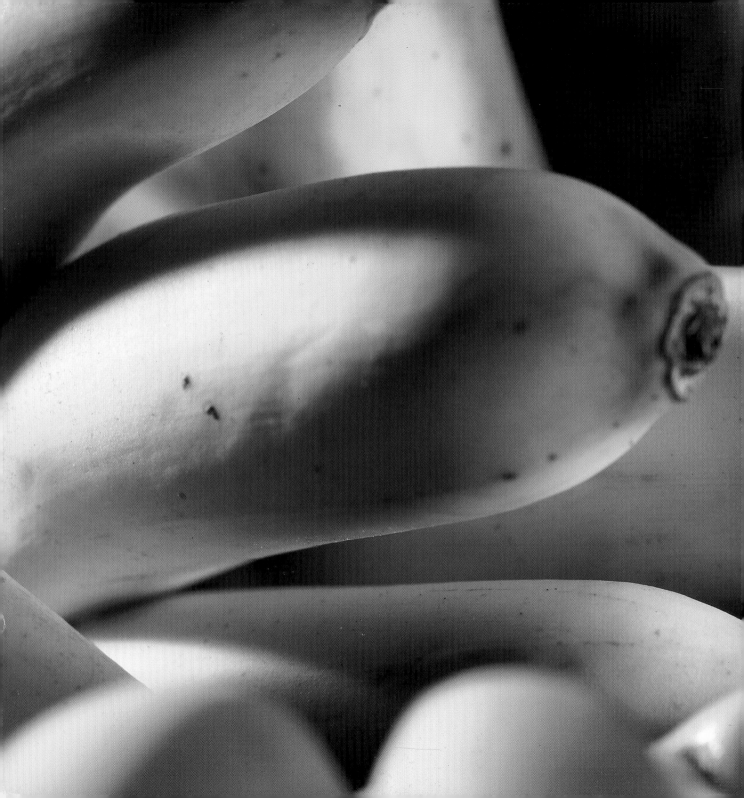

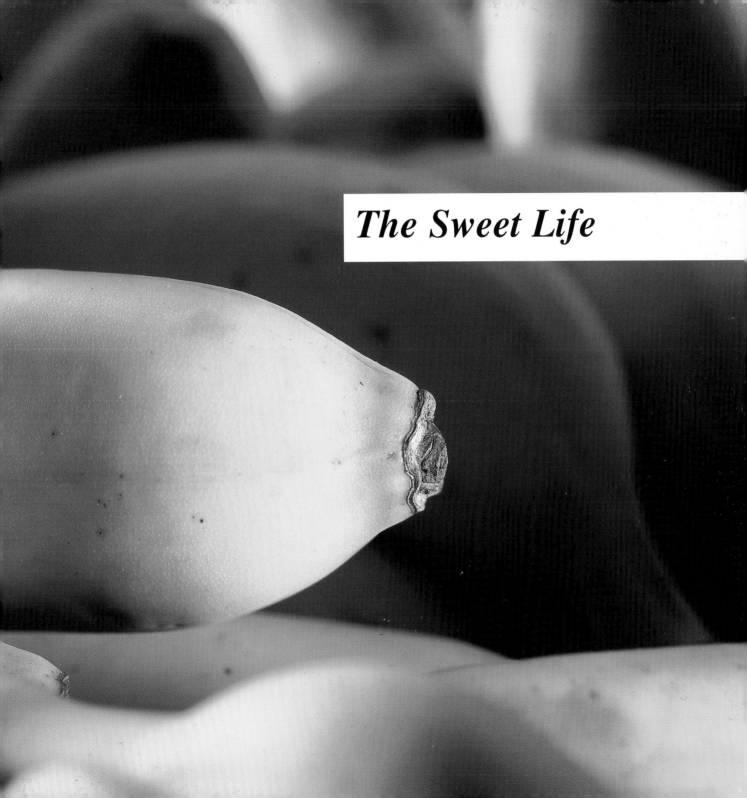

The Sweet Life

Sweet Dishes and Drinks

What You Should Drink

It is important to drink plenty of liquids, but not over ice or right out of the refrigerator. Cold beverages "put out" the digestive fire. Besides, drinking warm water is beneficial (see page 85), and, according to the Ayurveda, it belongs on every menu. Just try it once and you'll see!

Herb and spice teas, as well as Ayurveda coffee, also are recommended, depending on your taste and dosha dominance. Or, try hot water with a pinch of ginger or turmeric! Ayurveda coffee is a coffee substitute of herbs and exotic plants, and has a delicate bitter-coffee aroma and slight energizing effect. It does not have the stimulants and side effects of regular coffee (see ordering address on page 39).

Freshly squeezed fruit juices give immediate energy—the emphasis should be on "freshly squeezed." Fresh juice provides the body with more energy than is used in the digestion of them. Alcohol, on the other hand, upsets all three doshas.

Milk and Lassi

In the Ayurveda, milk is not so much a drink, as it is a whole meal. It should not be drunk with the meal, because the combination is indigestible. Preferably, milk should be drunk boiled, so that it is more easily digested. You can sweeten it according to your taste, or spice it with cardamom, ginger, cinnamon, anise, etc. When milk is digestible, it is the ideal fortifying between-meal snack.

Lassi, a yogurt drink (see page 93), is recommended regularly with meals, or for between-meal snacks.

The Desire for Something Sweet

The "sweet" taste (see page 57) is considered fundamental in the Ayurveda, since it promotes structure and growth and has a relaxing effect. Basic foods like grains, milk products, oil, fat, and sweeteners fall into the "sweet" category.

If you often crave something sweet, then your body is telling you that you need a sweet rasa now. Whether or not this need is produced by poor eating habits or bad nutrition, there are healthy ways to satisfy the need.

Chocolate produces large quantities of waste and generates ama. Instead of chocolate, have warm apple strudel; a cup of hot milk with some almonds; or a mixture of almonds, raisins, and a cookie. Also, a salad of ripe, sweet fruit is recommended. Dates and figs will satisfy this craving as well.

Sweeteners

• Refined sugar should be used only in small quantities. It is true that sugar will boost energy, but only for a short time; it eventually leads to an energy deficiency since, in the complex metabolic process, it has the effect of an "energy robber."

• We recommend that you sweeten foods with jaggery, unrefined cane syrup, maple syrup, pear nectar, or molasses, depending on the dosha dominance and taste (see tables on the back flap).

Jaggery—is a dark, coarse, unrefined sugar (sometimes referred to as palm sugar), and can be made from the sap of various palm trees or from sugar-cane juice. It comes in several forms, the two most popular being a soft,

honey-butter texture and a solid cake-like form. It can be purchased in East Indian markets.

• Honey also is sweet, but it has a predominantly tart taste. Therefore, honey is the only suitable sweetener for Kapha dominance. Honey should be bought cold-extracted, and never should be heated over 104° F (40° C). This follows the teaching in the Ayurveda that when honey is heated over 104° F (40° C), it becomes toxic and produces ama.

Sweet Foods

In the Ayurveda, one does not eat sweet foods as dessert after the main meal, but before or between meals, for instance, about 4 P.M. At this time, the Vata is at its highest, and something sweet is relaxing and settling.

How well you digest sweet things depends on when you eat them, and if you have a well-functioning digestive fire that will completely break down the food. If your digestive fire is weak, the food will not be digested properly, and waste products will be formed. Sweet foods are, therefore, not appropriate for people with weak digestion or Kapha dominance.

Ayurveda Tip : Warm Water

Drink warm water regularly! This quenches thirst, cleanses the sense of taste, and regulates the digestive fire. Boil filtered or spring water for at least 10 minutes over low heat in an open pot; boiling the water only a short time does not have the same effect. The longer it boils, the "finer" and "softer" it becomes, making it easier for the water to purify the body of waste products. Pour the water into a new thermos bottle, which will eliminate the possibility of residual flavors. Drink it at meals and in between.

To cleanse your system, drink a few swallows of water every 30 minutes for 2 weeks; how much water you drink matters less than the regularity in which you drink.

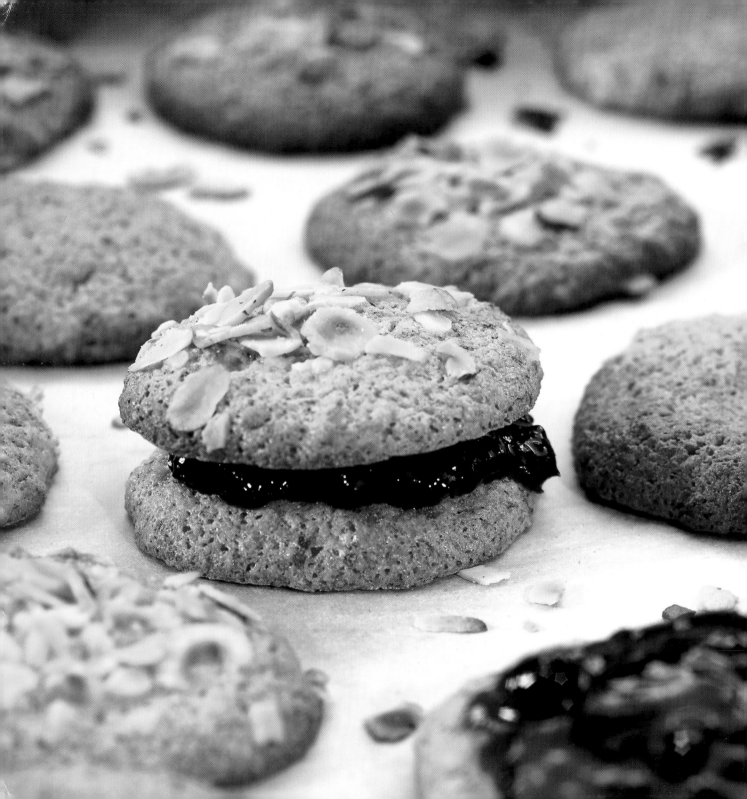

Fruit Doughnuts

Suitable for guests

• In a large bowl, stir the flour, cinnamon and milk to a smooth batter. Let it stand for about 2 hours (don't put it in the refrigerator).

• Heat the ghee in a small pot. Clean the fruit and cut it into small pieces. Fold the fruit into the batter, a handful at a time, until the fruit is well covered with batter.

• Remove each piece of fruit from the batter, letting them drip, and then fry in the hot ghee for about 4 minutes until they are golden brown. Continue to follow this procedure with the rest of the fruit. Makes 6–8 pieces.

Harmonize your dosha dominance:
Vata Use bananas, pineapple, or apple.
Pitta Use apples, bananas, or cherries.
Kapha Not suitable.

Nut Duchess

Pictured

• In a small bowl, mix the flour, ground nuts, and cinnamon. In another bowl, beat the egg whites stiff, gradually adding the sugar. Fold the nut mixture and butter into the egg whites with a whisk.

• Preheat the oven to 425° F (225° C). Fill a pastry bag or cookie press with the batter. Line a baking sheet with parchment paper. Lay out silver-dollar-size rounds of batter onto parchment. Top half of the rounds with chopped nuts. Bake the cookies for 10 to 13 minutes. Let cool, then spread the plain cookies with jam; place the nut-topped cookies on top. Makes about 30 cookies.

Harmonize your dosha dominance:
Vata Instead of wild fruit jam, use plum or cherry jam.
Pitta Instead of the hazelnuts, top with flaked coconut; use cherry or plum jam.
Kapha Eat these in moderation. Instead, eat muffins made with roasted barley, buckwheat, or millet.

Fruit Doughnuts

1 scant cup (100 g) chickpea flour (see page 56)

1/2 teaspoon ground cinnamon

scant 1/2 cup (100 ml) warm milk

1 lb (200 g) fruit (see doshas)

For deep frying:
1 1/8 lb (500 g) ghee, or as needed

Preparation time:
about 50 minutes
(+ 2 hours rising time)

Nut Duchess

3 tablespoons (40 g) wheat flour

scant 1/2 cup (100 g) ground hazelnuts

1 teaspoon ground cinnamon

5 egg whites

1/4 cup plus 1 tablespoon (100 g) granulated sugar

2 tablespoons (30 g) melted butter

1/2 cup (100 g) chopped hazelnuts

4 tablespoons wild fruit jam (strawberry, blackberry, etc.)

For the baking tin:
Parchment paper

Preparation time:
35–40 minutes

PER SERVING:	181 CALORIES	
NUTRITIONAL INFORMATION		
Carbohydrate	25	g
Protein	5	g
Total fat	9	g
Cholesterol	23	mg
Sodium	15	mg
Fiber	4	g

PER SERVING:	53 CALORIES	
NUTRITIONAL INFORMATION		
Carbohydrate	4	g
Protein	1	g
Total fat	4	g
Cholesterol	2	mg
Sodium	55	mg
Fiber	.5	g

Deep-fried Bananas

$^1/_2$ teaspoon ground cinnamon

1 teaspoon ground anise

$^1/_2$ teaspoon each, ground: cardamom and ginger

1 pinch salt

1 scant cup (100 g) chickpea flour (see page 56)

$^1/_4$ cup plus 1 tablespoon (75 ml) water

2 ripe bananas

2 teaspoons cold-filtered honey

4 lemon balm leaves

For deep-frying:

$1^1/_8$ lb (500 g) ghee, or as needed

Preparation time:
about 30 minutes
(+ 1 hour rising time)

Applesauce

2 lb (1 kg) apples

juice of 1 lime

3 cups ($^3/_4$ l) water, divided

1 cinnamon stick

1 whole clove

2 sprigs mint

2 teaspoons sugar

Preparation time:
about 40 minutes

Deep-fried Bananas
Classic

• In a large bowl, mix the spices, salt, and chickpea flour. Add the water bit by bit, stirring, until a thick batter has formed. Let rest for about 1 hour.

• Heat the ghee in a pan or a deep-fryer (up to 325° F [160° C]). The fat is hot enough when you hold a wooden spoon in it, and little bubbles rise around it.* Peel the bananas and slice $^1/_2$ inch thick. Dip slices in the batter, letting excess drip off. Place coated slices in ghee and fry until brown and crispy; this may have to be done in batches. Let slices cool on a wire rack. When the bananas have cooled some, drizzle some honey over top. Cut the lemon balm into strips and sprinkle it over top.

*(Alternatively, measure the temperature with a candy thermometer.)

Harmonize your dosha dominance:
Vata Very suitable without variations.
Pitta Leave out honey, if you wish.
Kapha Not suitable. Choose fresh fruit.

PER SERVING:	364 CALORIES
NUTRITIONAL INFORMATION	
Carbohydrate 62	g
Protein 11	g
Total fat 15	g
Cholesterol 33	mg
Sodium 158	mg
Fiber 9	g

Applesauce
Pictured

• Quarter the apples, peel, and remove seeds. In a large bowl, combine the lime juice with 2 cups ($^1/_2$ l) water; add the apples, and let soak several minutes.

• Combine 1 cup ($^1/_4$ l) water and 1 cup ($^1/_4$ l) lime-water mixture in a pot. Chop the apples and add to pot. Add cinnamon stick, clove, and mint and bring to a boil. Let cook, stirring occasionally, until liquid has just about evaporated; stir in the sugar, and let stand for 5 minutes. Remove spices and mint.

Harmonize your dosha dominance:
Vata Very suitable without variations.
Pitta Prepare without lime juice and use very sweet, ripe apples.
Kapha Prepare without sugar. If you eat the applesauce lukewarm, you can stir in 1 teaspoon honey.

Tips:
The applesauce is best served lukewarm. Tart, firm apples make the applesauce especially flavorful.
For children: Add raisins before liquid has evaporated.

PER SERVING:	278 CALORIES
NUTRITIONAL INFORMATION	
Carbohydrate 73	g
Protein 8	g
Total fat 1	g
Cholesterol 0	mg
Sodium 3	mg
Fiber 9	g

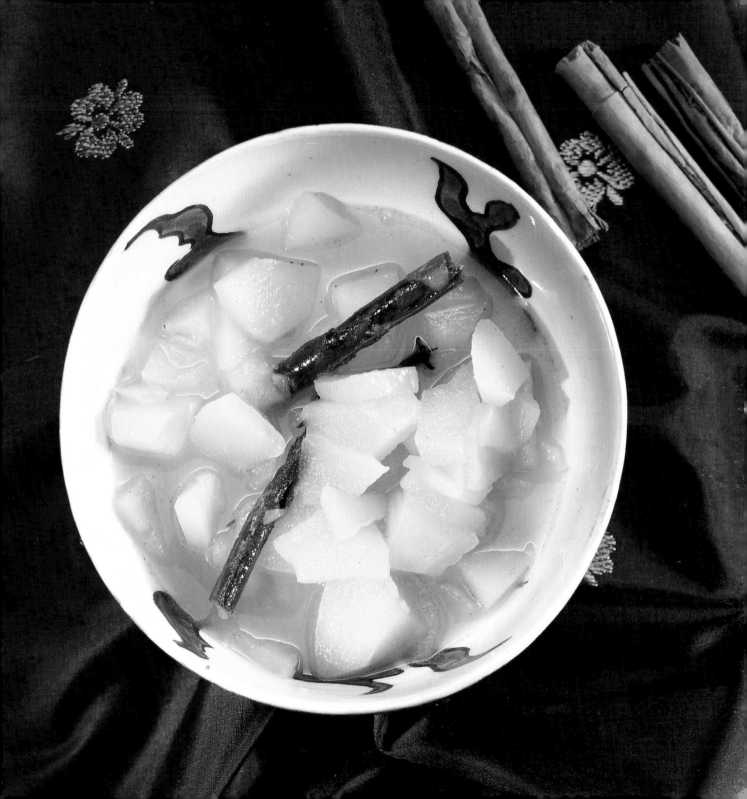

Nectar Rice Pudding

3 tablespoons (50 g) white
long-grain rice

4 cups (1 l) milk

1 or 2 bay leaves

2 tablespoons granulated
sugar or jaggery (page 85)

1/2 teaspoon ground cardamom

2 tablespoons sliced almonds

Preparation time:
about 50 minutes

Mango Ice Cream

1 small mango

scant 1/2 cup (100 ml) cream

1 teaspoon rose water
(available in health-food
stores and Asian markets)

ground cardamom to taste

1 teaspoon granulated sugar
or jaggery (page 85)

For garnishing as desired:

1 sprig lemon balm

pistachio nuts

Preparation time:
about 25 minutes
(+1 hour freezing time)

Nectar Rice Pudding
More time-consuming

• Rinse the rice and set aside. Put the milk in a large, heavy pot and let cook over low to moderate heat for about 20 minutes. Adjust the heat so the milk foams constantly without boiling over. Keep stirring while the milk thickens so it doesn't scorch on the bottom.

• Add the rice and bay leaves and keep stirring over low heat until the rice is tender.

• Add the sugar, cardamom, and almonds, and let cook 5 minutes more.

Harmonize your dosha dominance:
Vata Serve warm.
Pitta Add some rose water (available in health-food stores and Asian markets).
Kapha Not suitable.

Mango Ice Cream
Pictured

• Peel the mango; cut the flesh away from the pit and coarsely dice. Place mango, cream, rose water, cardamom, and sugar in the food processor; process to purée.

• Pour the mango mixture in a stainless steel bowl and place in the freezer for about 1 hour, stirring occasionally. Or, pour the mixture into the freezer cylinder of an ice-cream machine and freeze according to the manufacturer's instructions.

• To serve, cut the lemon balm leaves into strips and finely chop the pistachios. Scoop out the ice cream and serve with lemon balm strips and pistachios.

Harmonize your dosha dominance:
Vata Suitable in small amounts during summer.
Pitta Very suitable without variations.
Kapha Only a little during summer.

PER SERVING:	406 CALORIES	
NUTRITIONAL INFORMATION		
Carbohydrate	52	g
Protein	19	g
Total fat	14	g
Cholesterol	37	mg
Sodium	245	mg
Fiber	1	g

PER SERVING:	154 CALORIES	
NUTRITIONAL INFORMATION		
Carbohydrate	22	g
Protein	2	g
Total fat	7	g
Cholesterol	22	mg
Sodium	27	mg
Fiber	2	g

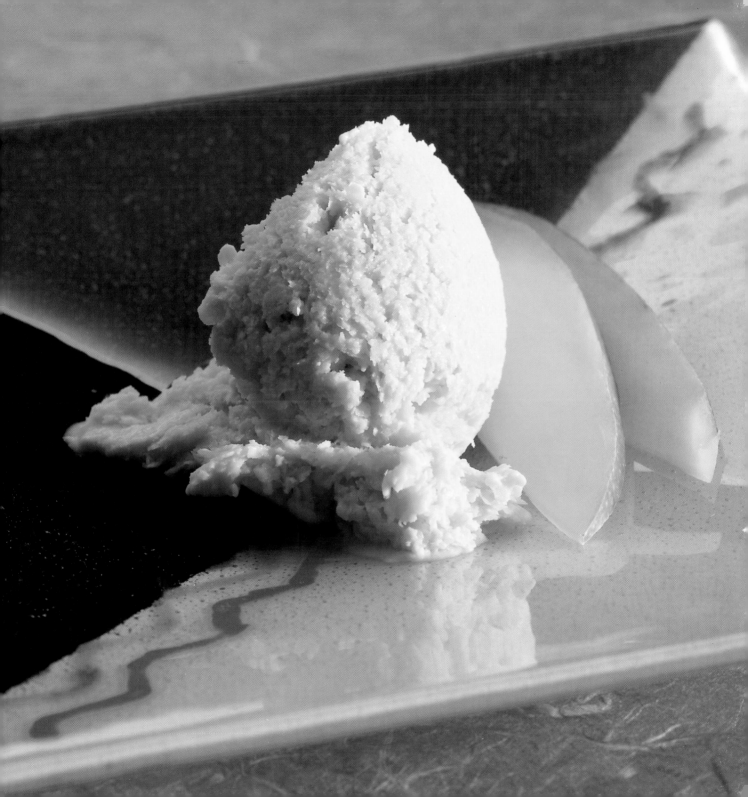

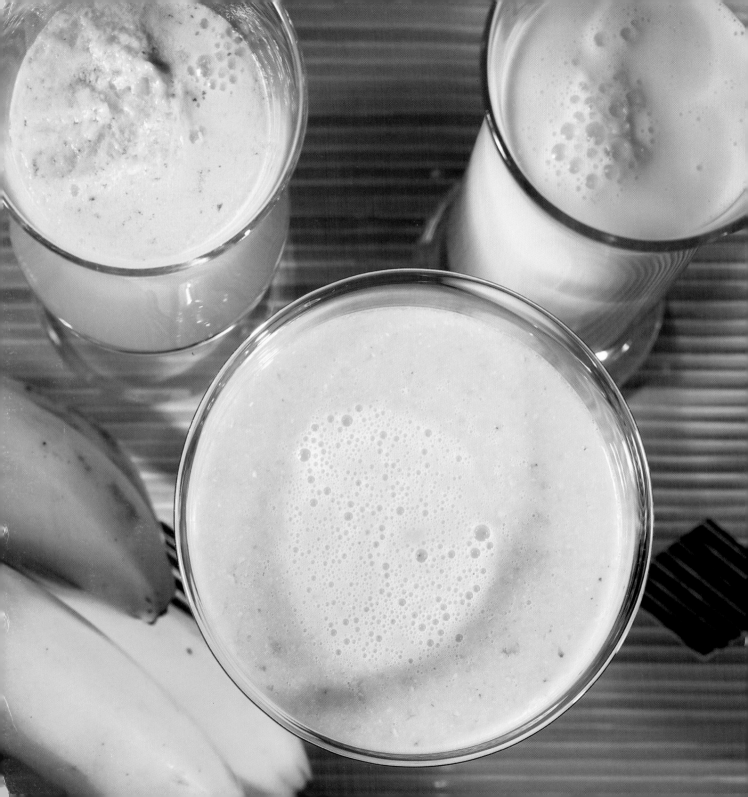

Drinks
Easy to prepare

Orange Shake

For 2 servings, cut 1 ripe banana into pieces and put in a blender. Add the juice of 6 oranges, 2 tablespoons flaked oats, 2 teaspoons lemon juice, 1 tablespoon mango pulp, and 1 teaspoon honey; process to purée. Divide shake between 2 glasses. Chop 6 cashews and sprinkle on top.

Harmonize your dosha dominance:
Vata Use very ripe, sweet fruit.
Pitta Instead of oranges, use sweet grapes (seedless or remove seeds) or grape juice. Leave out the lemon and honey.
Kapha Drink fresh apple juice or cider instead.

Avocado Cocktail

For 2 servings, dice 1 avocado and sprinkle it with the juice of 1 lime. Put it in a food processor and purée with the leaves of 2 dill sprigs and about 3½ tablespoons (50 ml) cream.

Divide mixture between 2 glasses, then fill with mineral water; season with salt, black pepper, and chili powder to taste.

Harmonize your dosha dominance:
Vata Don't drink too cold.
Pitta Use only a little lime juice. Add more fresh herbs, such as mint, dill, or cilantro.
Kapha Not suitable. Drink hot water (page 85) with pieces of fresh ginger.

Mango Lassi

For 1 serving, combine 2½ tablespoons mango purée, some cardamom, about ½ cup (125 ml) whole-milk yogurt and about ½ cup (125 ml) water in a blender; blend until the mixture is foamy and smooth. Pour into the glass and flavor with ½ teaspoon rose water (available in health-food stores and Asian markets).

Very suitable for all the doshas.

Pictured top left, Avocado Cocktail; top right, Orange Shake; and bottom, Mango Lassi.

Lassi—drink on a daily basis

This Ayurvedic yogurt drink is easily digestible, stimulates the appetite, is thirst-quenching, and stimulates digestion. It settles the stomach and, thus, is suitable for any dosha dominance. To make a lassi, start with homemade or store-bought fresh yogurt, then thin it with an equal amount of water. Beat the mixture with a wire whisk until it is smooth and foamy.

Lassi variations, add
- *cardamom, sugar, and rose water*
- *fresh mint and some salt*
- *ground ginger, cumin, and black pepper*
- *Mango Lassi (see recipe on this page)*

ORANGE SHAKE

PER SERVING:	330 CALORIES
NUTRITIONAL INFORMATION	

Carbohydrate	61	g
Protein	7	g
Total fat	8	g
Cholesterol	0	mg
Sodium	8	mg
Fiber	3	g

AVOCADO COCKTAIL

PER SERVING:	206 CALORIES
NUTRITIONAL INFORMATION	

Carbohydrate	15	g
Protein	3	g
Total fat	17	g
Cholesterol	10	mg
Sodium	164	mg
Fiber	9	g

MANGO LASSI

PER SERVING:	109 CALORIES
NUTRITIONAL INFORMATION	

Carbohydrate	13	g
Protein	5	g
Total fat	4	g
Cholesterol	14	mg
Sodium	56	mg
Fiber	.2	g

INDEX

U.S. Edition Copyright © 1997
Barron's Educational Series, Inc.

Published originally under the
title *Ayurveda Typgerecht Kochen*
Copyright © 1996 by Grafe und
Unzer Verlag GmbH, Munchen

*All inquiries should be
addressed to:*
Barron's Educational Series, Inc.
250 Wireless Boulevard
Hauppauge, New York 11788

International Standard Book No.
0-7641-0026-2

Library of Congress Catalog Card
No. 97-11041

Library of Congress Cataloging-
in-Publication Data

Bühring, Anne.
    [Ayurveda Typgerecht Kochen.
English]
    Auyrveda, cooking to suit your
body's needs / Anne Bühring,
Petra Räther ; photography,
Heinz-Josef Beckers.
        p.   cm.
    Includes index.
    ISBN 0-7641-0026-2
    1. Vegetarian cookery.
2. Medicine, Ayurvedic. I. Räther,
Petra. II. Title
RM236 IN PROCESS
641.5'636—dc21   97-11041
                               CIP

Printed in Hong Kong
987654321

Thanks to:
Josh Westrich and Christoph Fein
for their cooperation in
processing the photographs in
their photo studio in Essen.

Anne Bühring studied nutrition
and was a nutritional adviser for
self-help groups and in
environmental consulting. Since
1988, she has been a food editor
for some well-known magazines.
Since 1991, she has directed the
food department of a large
German health magazine.

Petra Räther is a trained
Maharishi Ayurveda health
consultant and meditation
teacher. She received her training
at the Maharishi European
Research University (MERU) in
Switzerland. Since 1989, she has
conducted courses and seminars
on the themes of Ayurveda and
meditation, primarily at the
Maharishi Ayurveda Health
Center in Hamburg.

Heinz-Josef Beckers studied
communications design at the
University of Essen (Folkwang).
He works with food, still life, and
experimental photography, as well
as graphic design for businesses,
publishers, and agencies.

Elizabeth D. Crawford is
responsible for the translation
from German.

The following tables offer a simple overview of the foods that help balance Vata, Pitta, and Kapha dominances. This compilation should be used as a reference, but is not set in stone. Listen to yourself! Your body knows exactly what it needs. You will find that much of what is suitable for you in the tables will appeal to your tastes anyway.

You will find even more information in the test interpretations of each dosha beginning on page 12.

Suitable Foods for Vata Dominance

General	Mainly sweet, sour, and salty foods. Warm foods and drinks preferred.
Vegetables (boiled)	Asparagus, beets, carrots, cucumbers, green beans, okra, batatas (sweet potatoes), radishes
(prepared with fat, in moderation)	Celeriac, celery, peas, potatoes, zucchini, tomatoes, green leaf vegetables, lettuce
Fruit (sweet and ripe)	Grapes, mangos, bananas, avocados, melons, papayas, berries, cherries, coconut, fresh figs, fresh dates, oranges, peaches, nectarines, pineapples, plums
Grains	Wheat—pasta, bread, farina (cooked) Oats—bread, rolled oats (cooked) Rice—basmati, whole-grain rice
Legumes	Yellow and green mung beans, red lentiles, chickpeas, tofu (in small quantities)
Milk products (all recommended, such as)	Milk, butter, cream, ghee, fresh cheese, lassi
Oil (all recommended, such as)	Sesame oil, sunflower oil, olive oil
Nuts and seeds (all in small amounts, such as)	Almonds (blanched), sesame seeds, cashews, sunflower seeds, pumpkin seeds
Sweeteners (all natural sweeteners, such as)	Jaggery, maple syrup, pear nectar, refined sugar, honey, rock candy (small amounts), molasses
Spices and herbs (all recommended, such as)	Ginger, cumin, rock salt, black pepper, cinnamon, cardamom, caraway, clove, mustard seed, asafetida, anise, fennel, turmeric, fenugreek, bay, nutmeg, basil, oregano, marjoram, thyme, cilantro, Vata churnas